Psychedelics
and Mental Health

"Neuroscientist Irene de Caso shows how psychedelics, when used safely and appropriately, can lead to positive and lasting change. This is an important book for anyone interested in the science of psychedelic-assisted mental health treatment."

RICK DOBLIN, PH.D., FOUNDER AND PRESIDENT OF
THE MULTIDISCIPLINARY ASSOCIATION
FOR PSYCHEDELIC STUDIES (MAPS)

"Featuring illustrations, diagrams, and flowcharts, *Psychedelics and Mental Health* clearly guides the reader step-by-step along neuro-psychological pathways that have previously baffled ordinary, non-scientific readers. By making ideas clear to both the sciences and the humanities, this book bridges the 'two-cultures chasm.'"

THOMAS B. ROBERTS, PH.D., AUTHOR OF
MINDAPPS, THE PSYCHEDELIC FUTURE OF THE MIND,
AND *PSYCHEDELICS AND SPIRITUALITY*

Psychedelics and Mental Health

Neuroscience and the Power of Psychoactives in Therapy

Irene de Caso, Ph.D.

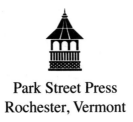

Park Street Press
Rochester, Vermont

Park Street Press
One Park Street
Rochester, Vermont 05767
www.ParkStPress.com

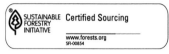

Text stock is SFI certified

Park Street Press is a division of Inner Traditions International

Copyright © 2022, 2025 by Irene de Caso

Originally published in 2022 as *Psychedelics and Mental Health: The Neuroscience Behind a New Psychotherapy* by Argonowta Digital SSL, Madrid, Spain

Note to the Reader: *This book is intended as an informational guide and should not be a substitute for professional medical care or treatment. Neither the author nor the publisher assumes any responsibility for physical, psychological, legal, or social consequences resulting from the ingestion of psychedelic substances or their derivatives.*

Cataloging-in-Publication Data for this title is available from the Library of Congress

ISBN 979-8-88850-000-2 (print)
ISBN 979-8-88850-001-9 (ebook)

Printed and bound in the United States by Lake Book Manufacturing, LLC
The text stock is SFI certified. The Sustainable Forestry Initiative® program promotes sustainable forest management.

10 9 8 7 6 5 4 3 2 1

Text design by Priscilla Baker and layout by Kenleigh Manseau
This book was typeset in Garamond Premier Pro with Arquitecta and Futura Std used as display typefaces

Creative Commons Agreements: CC BY 2.5: fig. 5; CC BY 3.0: fig. 38, fig. 41, plate 16, plate 19; CC BY-SA 3.0: fig. 26, fig. 50, fig. 56, plate 23; CC BY 4.0: fig. 18, fig. 47, fig. 54, plate 22; CC BY-SA 4.0: fig. 57, fig. 58; CC-BY-NC-ND 4.0: fig. 37.

To send correspondence to the author of this book, mail a first-class letter to the author c/o Inner Traditions • Bear & Company, One Park Street, Rochester, VT 05767, and we will forward the communication.

To those who boldly fight for our
right to cognitive liberty.

Contents

Foreword

José Carlos Bouso, Ph.D.

Jaques Monod, the Nobel laureate in Physiology or Medicine, took the quote attributed to Democritus: "Everything existing in the Universe is the fruit of chance and necessity," and applied it to the study of molecular biology and evolutionary models in his book *Chance and Necessity*. In the phrasing itself, the meaning is explained: It is the combination of chance and necessity that makes a phenomenon not just happen by chance, playing with infinite probabilities all the time, but something that is viable, for which necessity is required. This applies to many biological phenomena, but the expression also fits the case of some social phenomena. This is what is currently happening with what some call the "psychedelic renaissance" to refer to the renewed interest in hallucinogenic drugs in both popular and scientific circles. This phenomenon has been ongoing since the 1990s, when a relatively small group of scientists became interested in the pharmacology, neurobiology, and therapeutic potential of drugs classified as extremely dangerous because of their high abuse potential and lack of recognized medical properties and were, therefore, included in Schedule I of the 1971 United Nations Convention on Psychotropic Substances. Those scientists were from the United States (Rick Strassman, Manuel Tancer, and Charles Grob); Switzerland (Franz Vollenweider and Matthias Liechti);

Germany (Euphrosyne Gouzoulis-Mayfrank and Leo Hermle); and Spain . . . Spain? yes, Spain (Magí Farré, Jordi Riba, Jordi Camí, and Manel Barbanoj). The pioneering research of the 1990s was mainly carried out in Europe, even though the narrative about the psychedelic renaissance always refers to the Anglo-Saxon world. I'm talking about research with human beings, which is where the real difficulty arises. In fact, there were fewer than ten groups in the whole world doing this kind of research. These are the pioneers who are largely responsible for our being here now, but let's not get ahead of ourselves.

Since the 1990s, in parallel to this incipient interest in the scientific study of psychedelics, cultural interest has also been growing. Terence McKenna was a mass idol with his somewhat nonsensical but highly entertaining and even inspiring theories on almost every aspect of knowledge; and with him came a whole series of books and characters, each more fascinating than the next. It was the pre-internet era, and knowledge could only be obtained from books, scientific articles (if you were a university student) or lectures, which also proliferated during those years. Thus Jonathan Ott, Alexander Shulgin, and, of course, Albert Hofmann, invited by Antonio Escohotado and Josep Maria Fericgla, toured Spain and half the world. It is not in vain that Ott's *Pharmacotheon* and the Shulgins' *PiHKAL* and *TiHKAL* are the foundation stones of today's psychedelic edifice.

The symbiosis that exists between psychedelic science and popular culture can only be found in one other area of science: cannabis. Today, very few doctors know what the endocannabinoid system is, and many find it difficult to pronounce cannabidiol, let alone tetrahydrocannabinol, something that is in the everyday vocabulary of any cannabis user. The same goes for psychedelic science. Concepts such as default mode neural network or entropic brain (which de Caso will explain in the corresponding chapters of this book) are part of the everyday vocabulary of the average psychonaut. In 2010, as part of the psychedelic renaissance, a key organization called MAPS (Multidisciplinary Association for Psychedelic Studies) and its indefatigable founder, Rick Doblin, inaugurated the new era of psychedelic conferences, calling them "Psychedelic Science." Successive conferences have appeared not only in the United States (Horizons [perspectives on psychedelics] and queer psychedelics, for example), but also in the United Kingdom (the Breaking Convention [multidisciplinary conference on psychedelic consciousness]), Amsterdam (the ICPR [Interdisciplinary Conference on Psychedelic Research]), and Prague (Beyond Psychedelics [multidisciplinary conference on psychedelics])—to name just a few, as the list goes on and on. ICEERS (International Center for Ethnobotanical Education, Research, and Service), where I work, has already held three conferences exclusively on ayahuasca (Ibiza 2014, Rio Branco 2016, and Girona 2019), with a growing audience at each new one. The remarkable fact about these conferences is that they are conferences where the speakers are scientists, but the attendees are not necessarily so. Another singularity in the scientific world: There is no other field of science in which scientific conferences aimed at a general public are organized and also vastly successful. Regarding scientific production, something similar is happening. At the end of the 1990s, what was published on psychedelics in specialized scientific journals could be read in a few spare moments; nowadays, even for someone who works professionally in this field, as is my case, it is simply impossible to keep up with everything that is published. And the fact is that research on psychedelics is proving to be a kind of *strange attractor* for mainly a young public who, with the enthusiastic energy of youth, wants to make it their scientific career. And proof of this is the book you are now holding in your hands.

And so much for chance! To sum up, a series of unorganized and diverse cultural and scientific phenomena, each with its own trajectory, gradually gaining in popularity; the successive conferences held here and there; the rapid proliferation of information (not always accompanied by knowledge) offered by the internet; its associated music festivals, of course . . .; all of this converging in the second decade of the 21st century, where there exists a state of necessity for the phenomenon to become viable. The need could be summed up by the fact that prohibitionist drug policies have been a failure, and the population knows it, especially the young population. Biological psychiatry, based on psychopharmaceuticals, has failed. The harm has begun to become apparent, and pharmaceutical companies are withdrawing from psychopharmacological investment because not only are they not capable of innovating new drugs, but those that do exist have side effects that make them pay scandalous compensation. The media no longer focuses on the insanity and degradation produced by hallucinogens, but rather on their beneficial effects; and there is a new industry, led by the new billionaires, also attracted to these types of drugs, eager to invest in innovative medicines, willing to put up the money to transform all these drugs into medicines. Thus, chance and necessity have conspired, as they often do, so that in psychedelic science and culture, the future is already here.

Therefore, this book by Irene de Caso is like an immense gift, on the one hand, for those of us who are already beginning to find it difficult to keep updated and, on the other, for those who are approaching this field for the first time, so that they can update themselves on the state of the art of psychedelics-assisted psychotherapy, as well as the psychological and neurobiological processes that underpin it. If there has been a resurgence in psychedelic research, it has been as much about the interest in unraveling what these drugs do in the brain as it has been about how the experience can help people overcome their psychological problems. But even beyond that, it has been about how these drugs can benefit their personal well-being, their relationships with others, and their understanding of their own being, and their being in the world. Yes, paradoxically, if there is one thing that these so-called hallucinogenic drugs do well, it is to enable us to better understand the nature of reality. This is why they have been essential for the construction of the cosmovisions of so many Indigenous communities that customarily use them, precisely for that: to know. Substances such as psilocybin, LSD (lysergic acid diethylamide), ketamine, DMT (dimethyltryptamine), MDMA (ecstasy), 5-MeO-DMT, ayahuasca, and salvinorin-A are gradually becoming part of the seasoned psychonaut and the avant-garde scientist's vocabulary. And soon, like aspirin or paracetamol, they will be part of the popular vocabulary too.

Irene de Caso has done the rigorous work of not only gathering and compiling all this research (if she had only done that, this book would have been just another literature review), but of explaining the literature review with an understandable language and a light writing that translates into a pleasant read. Most interesting, however, from my point of view, is her effort to translate the complex neuroscientific concepts into a phenomenological description in such a way that, whether we understand the complex neuroscientific concepts to a greater or lesser extent, we can certainly understand how they might relate to the different phenomenological aspects often present during the psychedelic experience.

If you want to learn with an introduction to neuroscience, update your concepts with the most recent research, know what the state of research in psychotherapy with psychedelics is, and, especially and most importantly, what this research is for: this is your book.

Psychedelic drugs reveal our cognitive, emotional, and experiential functioning, hence their name, psychedelic ("mind unveiling"). To know how these drugs work is, in short, to know oneself better, so let us welcome this book!

JOSÉ CARLOS BOUSO, PH.D.,
SCIENTIFIC DIRECTOR OF ICEERS

JOSÉ CARLOS BOUSO is a clinical psychologist with a Ph.D. in pharmacology. He developed his scientific activities while at the Universidad Autónoma de Madrid, the Instituto de Investigación Biomédica IIB-Sant Pau de Barcelona, and the Instituto Hospital del Mar de Investigaciones Médicas de Barcelona (IMIM). During this time, he developed studies about the therapeutic effects of MDMA (ecstasy) and psychopharmacological studies on the acute and neuropsychiatric long-term effects of many substances, both synthetic and of plant origin. As the Scientific Director of ICEERS, the International Center for Ethnobotanical Education, Research, and Service, José Carlos coordinates studies on the potential benefits of psychoactive plants, principally cannabis, ayahuasca, and ibogaine, with the goal of improving public health. He is coauthor of numerous scientific papers and several book chapters. He is also a member of the Medical Anthropology Research Center (MARC) at the Universitat Rovira i Virgili in Tarragona, visiting professor in the mental health program at the Faculty of Medicine of the University of São Paulo in Riberão Preto, Brazil, and vice-president of the Society of Clinical Endocannabinology (SEC).

Unlocking the Therapeutic Power of Psychedelics

How does one begin writing a book? I close my eyes and take a deep breath, feeling that silent inner core whose existence I ignored a few years ago. And I wonder, would I have ever discovered it had I never tried psychedelics? I doubt it. How can someone start searching for something if they don't know it exists?

Now that mindfulness and meditation have reached the mainstream in the West, many people are discovering that other way of being and feeling, that inner core, through these avenues. However, at least on this side of the planet, this phenomenon was, undoubtedly, sparked by the countercultural movement of the 1960s brought about by the recreational use of LSD. Even today, when most people have already heard about meditation, many, myself included, only began to understand its value after having lived the psychedelic experience.

Suddenly, spiritual clichés previously devoid of meaning make perfect sense. One clearly understands the oneness of humanity and that of the holy whole. And, by sharpening the sensations related to breathing, paying attention to the present moment, and slowing down the inner dialogue, one obtains a deep and unimaginable peace. But unlike meditation, through which achieving such a revelatory experience usually

1

requires years of practice, with psychedelics it is often just a matter of taking the right dose in the right environment.

It is not surprising that experiences of this nature have the potential to bring about psychological well-being. However, as we shall see, this is not always the case. Unlike meditation, the psychedelic experience also has the potential to promote high levels of anxiety, intense panic, and even psychotic breaks, especially when abused or conducted in the wrong environment. As with so many other decisions in life, it all comes down to assessing the risk-benefit balance and acting responsibly. And, it is my opinion that, for many people, the benefits outweigh the risks.

A Mental Health Crisis

Despite the fact that famines have all but disappeared in the West, there's easy access to clean water, and death from disease and violence has been drastically reduced, there is no doubt that Western society is facing a serious mental health crisis. According to the INE (the Spanish National Institute of Statistics), ten people per day were already committing suicide in Spain before the pandemic—ten times more than the number of deaths due to traffic accidents!

Trauma, loneliness, and chronic stress. And a profound lack of meaning. Millions of people live kidnapped by their emotions. Possessed by them, some would say. Unable to be the masters of their behavior. We all experience this to a greater or lesser extent, but, why are some more resilient and able to better regulate their emotions than others? What is it that human beings require to heal their wounds and enjoy a life full of meaning?

The many available anxiolytics, antidepressants, psychotherapeutic techniques, and even the newly arrived and welcomed mindfulness practices, do not seem to be enough. Despite their undeniable utility, these tools seem to be failing for a disturbingly large number of people. Psychotherapy is expensive and time consuming, and psychotropic drugs often have unpleasant side effects. What is more, even in the absence of side effects and with time and money at their disposal, many patients are still unable to free themselves from a constant sense of deep fear and suffering. Could highly stigmatized substances associated with the world of nighttime debauchery be the new tool we so desperately need?

As we shall see, this may indeed be the situation we find ourselves in. But what substances are we referring to exactly? How should they be used? What psychopathologies could be treated with such molecules? How do they work?

Throughout this book, we will focus on two types of persecuted substances whose research in psychotherapeutic settings has exploded in the last decade: classic psychedelics, such as LSD, psilocybin, and DMT (commonly known as hallucinogens); and the empathogen MDMA (commonly known as ecstasy), which is considered an atypical or pseudopsychedelic.

The Discovery, Prohibition, and Rebirth of New Tools in Psychotherapy

Nowadays most ordinary citizens associate substances such as LSD, magic mushrooms, and the famous ecstasy, with recreational environments. Although more and more people are becoming aware of their therapeutic applications, very few know that it was within a clinical setting where they first appeared. However, they eventually escaped from the laboratories and entered the world of leisure, which culminated in their subsequent illegalization and stigmatization. It is for this reason that the recent return of these substances to the research institutions is being called "the psychedelic renaissance," given that there was already extensive research into their psychotherapeutic potential in the past. With the advent of the Controlled Substances Act and the beginning of the war on drugs, promoted by Nixon in the early 1970s, such research was, however, abruptly halted and the regulatory agencies of the time placed both molecules (first LSD and later MDMA) in the Schedule I category (the same category as heroin!). This is where substances supposedly devoid of medical use, considered dangerous even under supervision, and having a high potential for abuse, are placed. Why were they placed here?

Such classification was mainly motivated by political and social reasons rather than based on medical evidence. The psychedelic experience was leading young people to demonstrate against the Vietnam War and the materialistic culture, revolutionizing American society, and threatening the social order of the time. It would, however, be unfair to ignore that the careless use of psychedelics was spreading throughout the youth, causing frequent accidents and traumatic experiences in users. Nevertheless, studies carried out with LSD and MDMA under controlled settings were pointing to an important medical potential that was, either intentionally or accidentally, ignored by the legislators when they decided to classify them into the Schedule I category. But let's not get ahead of ourselves and instead return to the beginning of these molecules' fascinating discovery.

Lysergic acid diethylamide, known as LSD, was first synthesized by the chemist Albert Hofmann in 1938. At the time, Hofmann was working for Sandoz, a pharmaceutical company based in Basel, Switzerland. They were trying to find a treatment for migraines, searching for molecules with vasostimulant properties in ergot (a fungus that infects rye). However, animal studies revealed no effects, other than a certain behavioral agitation, so further research was discontinued.

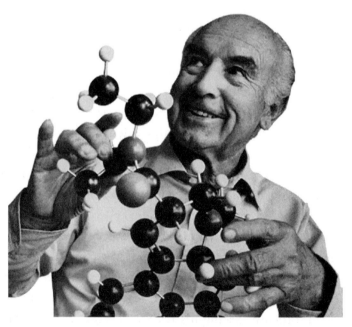

Albert Hofmann holding a representation of LSD's molecular structure.

However, for some mysterious reason, five years later this molecule was still present in the chemist's mind, as he had a "peculiar presentiment" that the molecule hid some interesting properties. In retrospect, he recounts how it was not he who chose LSD but LSD who "found" him and "called" him. On April 16, 1943, he proceeded to repeat his synthesis, despite Sandoz having a strict policy against resuming research with substances that had been previously discarded.

It was during the last synthesis processes that Hofmann began to feel the first unusual sensations. A certain agitation and dizziness seized his body, forcing him to interrupt his work and go home to rest. Once there, lying on the sofa, he began feeling a certain intoxication, which he described as not unpleasant. On closing his eyes "an uninterrupted stream of fantastic pictures, extraordinary shapes with intense, kaleidoscopic play of colours" occupied his mind, eventually concluding that he must have absorbed a small amount of the substance he'd been working with.

Intrigued as to how a molecule could have such a powerful psychoactive effect, three days later he ventured to take 0.25 mg in a controlled manner under the supervision of his laboratory assistant. Such an experimental dose was seemingly minuscule. However, we now know that it corresponded to a very high dose of LSD, the usual dose being about 125 micrograms. Hofmann was about to experience the first LSD trip in history. After forty minutes, he began to feel the first effects, which he describes in his laboratory notebook as "dizziness, feeling of anxiety, visual distortions, symptoms of paralysis, desire to laugh," these being the first and last notes he was able to take on that historic day.

Frightened by the intensity of the experience, he asked his assistant to accompany him home. Since it was wartime and transportation by car was forbidden, he used his bicycle. From then on, April 19 has become a day of celebration within the psychedelic community, known as Bicycle Day, and the bicycle, a representative icon of LSD.

No wonder this first LSD trip, not only given its potency but also given the absolute lack of knowledge regarding its toxicity, was terrifying for Hofmann. Seeing his reality drastically transformed and his volition vanished, he believed he had gone hopelessly insane, as if

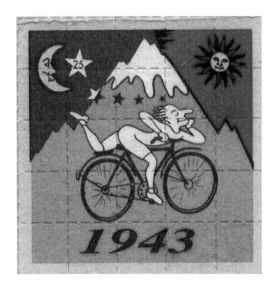

LSD sheet. Each of the squares bounded by the dotted line represents an LSD tab. The lysergic sheets often present a drawing, in this case, a cartoon of Dr. Hofmann riding his bicycle.

possessed by a demon. His assistant called a doctor who measured his vital signs and found nothing unusual other than an excessive dilation of the pupils and, gradually, he returned to ordinary reality. Imagine his relief as the danger of insanity faded away! As he enjoyed the still present visual effects, the feelings of terror were replaced by a profound sense of fortune and gratitude. He finally managed to sleep, and, when waking up the next day, he felt splendid, perceiving the vibrant world "as if newly created."

Suspecting that this potent substance might have important value in psychiatry, Hofmann quickly contacted other researchers. This time taking a third of the dose ingested by Hofmann, they repeated his experiment and were astonished. Soon, a new line of research was initiated.

As we will see further on, the psychedelic experience has certain properties that made LSD a great candidate as a psychotherapeutic tool. Therefore, after demonstrating its extremely low toxicity through animal experimentation, researchers proceeded to study its use in humans. One of the pioneering psychiatrists using this molecule was Humphry Osmond, who coined the term psychedelic, referring to the ability these types of substances have to manifest or expand (*delos*) the contents of the psyche (*psyque*).

In the 1950s, multiple studies were carried out with LSD. Particularly notorious were those aimed at treating alcoholism. Clinics started appearing that simultaneously administered LSD to several people who could, afterwards, meet to discuss their experiences. The results were promising. However, many of the studies of the time have been criticized for not having followed a rigorous methodology.[1] To tackle this issue, Krebs and Johansen conducted a meta-analysis,[2] published in 2012, that focused only on those studies that met the standards required today. The results revealed that, out of five hundred thirty-six participants, 59 percent of the participants in the group taking LSD significantly decreased their alcohol consumption, compared to only 38 percent within those in the placebo-administered control group. These results suggested that, when it comes to treating addictions, LSD does indeed have some psychotherapeutic potential. In the coming chapters, we will see how recent studies using psychedelic-assisted therapy seem to support this.

The same properties that made LSD an extraordinary molecule in psychotherapy soon attracted the attention of people outside the medical environment, causing an epidemic of consumption in the population. This epidemic was largely promoted by two professors of psychology at Harvard University: Timothy Leary and Richard Alpert, who, after experiencing LSD's effects, became its apostles. They undoubtedly played a key role in initiating the countercultural revolution of the 1960s, which was characterized by an explosion of creativity, but also by a cascade of accidents and psychic problems due to its irresponsible use. Hofmann's initial sense of satisfaction eventually turned into concern, leading him to write *LSD: My Problem Child*, a book where he carefully recounts his famous first LSD trip, his iconic bicycle ride, and the events that followed his historical discovery. In 1962, the authorities began to persecute the molecule and, in 1965, Sandoz finally halted its production.

---

1. A rigorous methodology, for example, consists of carefully controlling all variables to which participants are exposed; having a control group that has not taken any substances, with which to compare the results of the experimental group; and that neither the participants nor the researchers know which experimental group the participant belongs to.
2. A meta-analysis is a statistical analysis that combines the results of many similar studies.

Something similar occurred with MDMA a little later. MDMA (3,4-methylenedioxymethamphetamine) was first synthesized by Merck Pharmaceuticals in 1912 while searching for drugs capable of controlling bleeding. In the absence of the desired effects, research was eventually abandoned. It was not until the mid-1970s when, in the pursuit of psychoactive molecules with psychotherapeutic potential, chemist Alexander "Sasha" Shulgin decided to experiment with this molecule on himself. He immediately became convinced of its therapeutic potential. In addition to MDMA, Shulgin created a whole collection of psychoactive molecules and he, his wife Ann, and a group of close students ingested each one of them and described their effects in detail. Such "trip reports" can be found in *TiHKAL* and *PiHKAL*, two famous books written by the couple.

In the late 1970s, Shulgin introduced the MDMA molecule to Leo Zeff, who had been leading the underground psychedelic-assisted psychotherapy movement since LSD's prohibition. At that time, MDMA was still legal, promising to be a potent psychotherapeutic tool; but, like LSD, it ended up becoming popular within leisure environments. As its use shifted from a medicinal to a recreational setting, in 1984, the DEA (the American Drug Enforcement Administration) placed

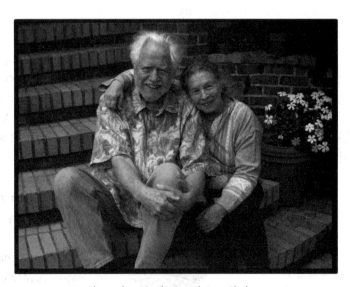

Alexander "Sasha" and Ann Shulgin.

this substance, along with LSD, in Schedule I, together with the most persecuted molecules. Such a decision was based on the relatively high abuse potential that this substance was proving to have but completely ignored the psychotherapeutic developments that were being achieved.

The psychotherapeutic potential of substances that were proving to be successful within clinical settings was shamefully ignored by the authorities, who instead banned the ongoing research and, harshly and unjustly, began to prohibit the substances. Thanks to the relentless efforts of people like Amanda Feilding, founder of the Beckley Foundation, who played a key role in funding the initial research and disseminating the substances' benefits from an early stage; and Rick Doblin, founder of MAPS (the Multidisciplinary Association for Psychedelic Studies), a nonprofit organization that since prohibition of LSD has been pressuring government regulatory agencies and funding a multitude of studies and conferences, the research was finally resumed after two decades. We can't thank them enough for their magnificent and historic work!

Throughout their respective organizations, Amanda and Rick managed to find researchers at universities (some as prestigious as London Imperial College and Johns Hopkins University) to carry out studies, not only on the clinical potential of psychedelics, but also on their effect on normal brain functioning.

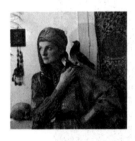

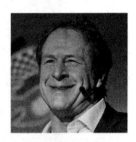

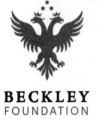

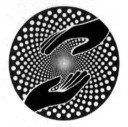

Amanda Feilding on the *left* and Rick Doblin on the *right,* along with the logos of their respective organizations: the Beckley Foundation and the Multidisciplinary Association for Psychedelic Studies, known as MAPS.

As we will see in chapter 2, the clinical results obtained in these initial studies were quite promising, drawing the attention of the media, patients, mental health professionals, and researchers, as well as the attention of philanthropists and investors. Rick, Amanda, and the pioneering scientific experts who accompanied them had sparked the "psychedelic renaissance," which has produced an exponential growth of scientific publications and, by 2021, brought the psychedelic substance market to a value of $487.5 million U.S. For a more in-depth reading regarding the fascinating history of psychedelic substances, I recommend a forthcoming book *The Psychedelic Reawakening* by Antón Gómez-Escolar.

This book will focus on reviewing the clinical studies that reveal the promising psychotherapeutic potential of psychedelics, describing their subjective effects, and explaining how they might be interacting with the brain and altering its behavior.

To ease the understanding of this last goal, I thought it necessary to begin with an introductory chapter on neuroscience. In this chapter, we will first study the anatomy and functioning of a neuron (receptors, neurotransmitters, action potentials, etc.). We will also learn how, in order to allow for a conscious experience to emerge, the information gathered by the senses is integrated, focusing on the essential role played by the thalamus (a subcortical structure), the cerebral cortex, and the required information-encoding processes. We will also study the way in which our decisions are guided by our fears and desires and how cortical activity is organized into functional networks. In addition to this chapter, you can also find "References for Further Study" at the end of each chapter and an extensive glossary at the end of the book. I hope that relevant concepts will be well understood and easy to access when we embark on the scientific theories regarding how these substances alter ordinary states of consciousness and why such alterations may have therapeutic effects. Readers with advanced knowledge of neuroscience can skip the chapter called "Understanding Neuroscience" if they wish, while those new to the topic can easily return to it as concepts reappear in future chapters. I hope that you will enjoy this journey, traveling with me from the inner world of a neuron all the way up to human behavior!

A warning is needed before we delve deeper into this material. Although neuroscience is undoubtedly advancing, we still have many more questions than answers. Despite this, even if only in a limited and reductionist way, we are gradually approaching a more accurate, or at least more detailed, version of that which we did not know before. Where only a vacuum of knowledge existed before, a new universe of data, theories, and, of course, new questions is now emerging. As we will appreciate throughout the book, and as anyone can intuitively imagine, the complexity we face when trying to study the brain and, more specifically, the brain-mind relationship, is practically infinite. Imagine adding mental health to this already complicated dyad! Therefore, I would like to caution you that the information presented in this book, particularly that related to the mechanisms of action of these substances, offers only theories. As such, they will be subject to change as research progresses. We will often have to engage in an intensive speculative exercise, especially when interpreting the neuroimaging results. This is the only way in which science can advance when the field we are studying is as deeply complex and unknown as the brain!

Having said that, I hope to be able to convey, in a clear and accurate manner, the knowledge I have accumulated over the years about how psychedelics alter the dynamic organized activity of the brain and some thoughts on how this disruption of information processing explains different aspects of the psychedelic phenomenology. Importantly, we will also explore how phenomenological aspects of these altered states might be contributing to their transformative and therapeutic potential. I feel compelled to emphasize this last word: potential. As enthusiastic as I might sound throughout the book, a therapeutic transformation after a psychedelic experience is not something that one should always expect. These experiences can be highly unpredictable and not something to be taken lightly, particularly in the case of classic psychedelics. These substances can reveal the fragility of the psyche's stability and abruptly shift the way we perceive ourselves and everything around us, which can lead down paths of confusion. Nonetheless, the extensive collection of second-hand accounts reported by users, the nascent clinical results in the existing modern literature, and the little first-hand experience that I have personally gathered, make me believe that these molecules do truly have a transformative potential. A potential that is certainly worth further exploration, because endless questions on how to harness it still remain to be answered. Importantly, as we will explore throughout the book, given these molecules' profound yet reversible effects on consciousness, they offer a unique and powerful research tool capable of helping us disentangle the brain's deepest mysteries.

References for Further Study

Hofmann A, Ott J. 1980. LSD, My problem child (Volume 5). New York (NY): McGraw-Hill.

Shulgin Alexander, Shulgin Ann. 1992. PiHKAL: A chemical love story. Berkeley (CA): Transform Press.

Shulgin Alexander, Shulgin Ann. 1997. TiHKAL: The continuation (Volume 546). Berkeley (CA): Transform Press.

1

Understanding Neuroscience

Before we delve into this chapter, I must warn you. Its content is rather technical and contains years of study condensed into a few pages. By the end, you will have acquired a fairly deep understanding of how the brain has evolved to perceive, feel, and act.

To achieve this, we must first descend into the inner world of the neuron and then zoom out to study how information is integrated in order to give rise to our rich conscious experience, with all the internal and external perceptions that exist within it: images, sounds, sensations, thoughts, emotions, and so on.

It will not always be an easy read, as it will entail studying the complex neuroanatomical circuits between different brain regions. This way, in later chapters, you'll be able to understand the implications surrounding the neuroimaging results obtained in psychedelic research. But don't despair! You will be accompanied by a multitude of visual resources at all times aimed at significantly easing your understanding.

Please also note that when in later chapters we allude to the information presented here, the relevant facts will be repeated more concisely. When necessary, you will also be redirected to the relevant figures and sections within this chapter to help you refresh your memory.

What I wish to convey with this warning is that the path we will follow in this chapter will give you a relatively detailed overview of how the brain works—a fascinating task, and by no means a trivial one! As you read on, don't worry about retaining all the information presented here. There will be plenty of opportunities to later review it. And above all, don't give up! I promise you that the next chapters will not be as technical.

If you still find it too challenging, you can always skip it and go to the lighter chapters ahead, returning here only when you need to review specific concepts mentioned further on. Maybe, once you are trapped by the wonders of the human mind, you will have the patience and inner drive to study it in detail.

That said, I encourage you not to succumb too easily and give it a try; so, grab a coffee, put on your nerdy glasses, and let's dive together into the electric and ingenious world of the nervous system. Are you ready?

Living Organisms: The Cell

Living organisms. What are they? What are we? Mostly, a bunch of rather common elements (e.g., oxygen, carbon, hydrogen, nitrogen, calcium, phosphorus) that anyone can easily buy, but it is not the elements alone that contain the value of life, but the way in which this elemental matter arranges itself—all thanks to the ability that atoms have, according to their particular properties, to bind with one another, which in turn allows them to form stable structures of higher order: molecules, which form cells, which form tissues, which form organs, which form complex pluricellular plants, fungi, and animals.

Some atoms can only bind to another atom, other atoms can bind to two atoms, and other atoms—like carbon—can bind to four different atoms. Let's look at an example: water. Water is made of many molecules of H_2O, meaning that each molecule of water is composed of an oxygen atom (O), and two hydrogen atoms. This is because oxygen atoms have two "hands," and hydrogen has one "hand," so the oxygen atom holds two hydrogen atoms, one with each hand, forming H2O, the molecule that makes up 62 percent of an adult human body. Water is contained inside a membrane—the cellular membrane. Here is where the magic of life and information processing begins: in the membrane. But first we must talk about the carbon atom.

Carbon atoms, and the stable bonds they form with hydrogen atoms, provide the backbone of most molecules that make up and are found in living organisms (i.e., biomolecules referred to as organic matter). Each carbon atom has four "arms" and in addition to binding to hydrogen atoms, they often use one or two (or even three) of their arms to bind to other carbon atoms, forming long chains, rings, and complex branched structures. Depending on the exact composition of these carbohydro-based molecules we can find several types of organic molecules within the cell: sugars, fats, proteins, and nucleic acid.[1] For example, fats make up the cellular membrane (see figure 1) and, in the watery space that they contain inside of them, you can find incredibly complex machinery comprising, among other structures, the nucleus, which houses the genetic code, elegantly encoded within the double helix of DNA (built from four different types of nucleic acid). This DNA molecule contains all the information needed to generate the proteins that make up the hardware of the body. So, when a protein needs to be synthesized, the sequence of DNA that contains "the recipe" for that specific protein is used as a template to produce a sequence of RNA. This small sequence of RNA is called messenger RNA (mRNA) (a concept with which you will have become familiar by

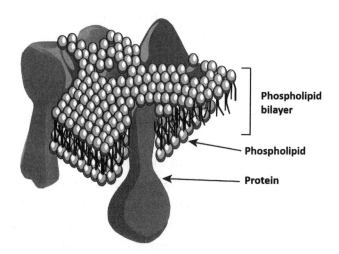

Figure 1. Phospholipid membrane with proteins embedded within it.

---

1. Nucleic acids are the building blocks of DNA and RNA molecules.

now if you have paid attention to the mechanism of action of the innovative Covid-19 vaccines), and will then be used for the synthesis of the specific protein for which it codes. In other words, the protein is generated from a messenger RNA sequence and the messenger RNA is generated from a small section of the DNA strand, whereby each section of DNA that codes for a specific protein is what we refer to as a gene.

Thanks to these genes, cells can synthesize many types of proteins, which serve diverse functions. Some of these proteins are used to catalyze chemical reactions involved in cellular metabolism, whereas others are located within the cellular membrane. Within the cellular membrane we can find proteins that act as selective channels, endowing the cellular membrane with a selective permeability, whereby certain ions can move in and outside of the cell; these channels can be open or closed depending on the signals that they receive from their internal and external environment.

Ultimately, cells are delimited by their membranes and consist of little aqueous organisms with dissolved ions (i.e., atoms that are charged positively or negatively) and other charged molecules such as proteins inside of them. Thanks to the cellular membrane's selective permeability, which is provided by the channels, the content inside the cell significantly differs from that of the extracellular space, whereby the interior of cells is more negatively charged than the exterior.

In addition to the channels, the cellular membrane also contains another very important type of protein: receptors. These proteins pierce through the membrane, so that one of their extremes is in touch with the external environment and the other with the internal one. Depending on the nature of the external section of the receptor, different molecules from the environment, such as drugs, can interact and bind to them, causing a conformational change in the receptor's structure, triggering an intracellular cascade of information that will signal a series of changes inside the cell.

The positive and negative charge levels inside human cells, including neurons (nerve cells), are mainly set by the concentrations of sodium ($Na+$), potassium ($K+$), chlorine ($Cl-$) and calcium ($Ca2+$) ions (i.e., atoms with positive or negative electrical charges), and fluctuate continuously thanks to the proteins located in the neuronal membrane that, by acting as ion channels, allow the passage of ions through the membrane (figure 2). Some of these channels only allow the passage of a particular type of ion (e.g., Na+) while others are less specific. Depending on the signals they receive from the environment, they will be open or closed, thereby modifying the balance between positive and negative ions inside the neuron. This movement of ions through the membrane will depend on the difference in concentration and charge between the inside and outside of the cell. If, for example, the sodium (Na+) channel is opened and the concentration of this ion is higher inside than outside the cell, the ion, moving in favor of its concentration gradient, will exit the neuron. But, in addition to the concentration gradient, this process also takes into account the charge difference between the interior and the exterior of the neuron. That is to say, if in addition to the difference in concentration, the outside is more negative than the inside, the sodium (Na+) will leave the cell even faster, since, in addition to the concentration gradient, the positive charge of this ion will be attracted by the negative charges on the outside. Instead, as the positive charge on the outside increases, and since charges of the same sign repel each other, the speed at which the Na+ exits the neuron will decrease. Thus, the direction in which the ions move across the membrane will be determined by simultaneously accounting for the difference in charge and concentration between the inside and outside of the cell. In more technical terms, the ions will pass through the membrane following an electrochemical gradient.

Ultimately, by creating a membrane which hosts channels and receptors, nature has created the building blocks of all life: the cell. An organism capable of interacting with elements outside of itself and recoding such external information into internal signals that promote changes within its internal space—changes that signal all sorts of intracellular responses to the detected stimuli such as the opening of channels or the expression of genes.

Living organisms, spanning from single cells to a full human body, exist in a dynamic equilibrium. This dynamic equilibrium is maintained through a variety of regulatory mechanisms collectively known as homeostasis. Thus, for the cells to properly respond to the signals in their external environment, and to trigger the intracellular cascade of information, their interior has to be in a particular state. When the cell responds to the signals from its environment, its internal state changes, becoming no longer able to respond to new signals, and so homeostatic mechanisms are needed to bring the cell back to its basal responsive state, with ion channels playing a key role in maintaining cellular homeostasis.

So far, we have looked at individual cells, but for some reason, cells decided to start working together to form pluricellular organisms.[2] Pluricellular organisms in most cases are formed by cells that contain the exact same DNA yet are tremendously different. How does this happen? How does an organism that contains the same DNA in all its cells show such complexity and heterogeneity?

After sperm has attached to an egg, cell division begins: two cells, four cells, eight cells, and so on. At first, all the cells are the same, but as they divide and the fetus develops, the cells that make up the fetus begin to differentiate. How can cells that were initially identical begin to differentiate from each other? They do so by expressing different genes contained within their DNA sequence, and by doing so producing different proteins. In other words, each cell generates different messenger RNAs from the DNA sequence that is common to all, thereby synthesizing different proteins that will give each cell its particular properties. This is how, through the production of different proteins and despite containing the same DNA, two cell types can end up forming tissues as different as, for example, skin (made up mostly of epithelial cells) or bone (made up mostly of bone cells). Or in the case that concerns us here, the nervous system, which is mostly made up of neurons.

The Neuron

There are many types of neurons, but, generally, they all tend to be asymmetrical cells. As we can see in figure 3, several projections emerge from the cell's main body (known as the soma), where the cellular nucleus is contained. Most of these projections are in charge of detecting signals

---

2. In order to learn more about why and how this happens, I urge you to study Michael Levin's groundbreaking work on bioelectrical networks.

present in the external fluid (neurotransmitters or drugs), and they do so thanks to numerous receptors located in their membranes.[3] These information-receiving projections are called dendrites.

One of the projections leaving the neuronal body is different from the dendrites. It is the axon, and it is in charge of sending the information that the dendrites pick up to other neurons. How does this happen? As we have seen, neurons, like other cells, are composed of water with dissolved ions inside of them, charged either positively or negatively. Under normal circumstances, when the neuron is in its baseline resting state, there is much more positive charge outside of the neuron than inside of it. However, when the receptors in the neuron's membrane get stimulated by an excitatory[4] molecule, they can trigger the opening of channels that allow positively charged ions to enter the neuron. This is key because when the positive charge inside the soma exceeds a certain threshold, an electric current is transmitted along this axonal projection. When the electric current (technically called an action potential) reaches the axon's terminal,[5] it triggers the production of neurotransmitters and signals their insertion into vesicles, as well as their subsequent release to the extracellular space (called the synaptic cleft).[6] The newly released neurotransmitters will then be detected by receptors located on the dendrites of the next neuron, and if the receptors in this following neuron receive enough stimulation, the neuron will fire an action potential transmitting the information to the following neuron.[7]

---

3. Specifically, receptors are located on small protrusions called synaptic boutons.

4. In contrast to inhibitory molecules, excitatory molecules promote changes inside the neuron that facilitate the firing of an action potential. Inhibitory molecules promote changes inside the neuron that impede the neuron from firing an action potential.

5. The transmission of this current is facilitated by the myelin sheath, a layer of flat cells that surrounds the axon acting as an insulating material.

6. The neurotransmitters are introduced into the vesicles via proteins located in the vesicles' membranes (in chapter 5 we will see how MDMA's mechanism of action involves these proteins), and the neurotransmitter's release takes place through the fusion of the vesicles' membranes with that of the axon terminal.

7. The neurotransmitter-mediated communication between the two neurons is what we refer to as a synapse (the neuron that releases the neurotransmitter is the presynaptic neuron, and the neuron that receives it is the postsynaptic neuron).

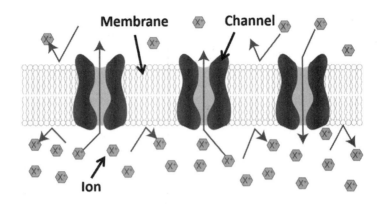

Figure 2. Ion channels located in the membrane through which ions enter or leave the neuron following their electrochemical gradient.

Other key proteins called neurotransmitter reuptake proteins (see figure 3) are anchored to the membrane of the axon terminal. These proteins are responsible for reintroducing the neurotransmitters from the synaptic cleft back into the axon terminal of the presynaptic neuron. Thus, not only are the neurotransmitters recycled so that they can be released again when another action potential is generated. These proteins also clear the synaptic cleft, ending the previous signaling. This way, the next time that the presynaptic neuron releases neurotransmitters, the receptors of the postsynaptic one will be available to receive the new signal.

After this overview of the neuron and the synapse, let's take a closer look at what causes the generation of an action potential in the first place. Let us repeat: when the positive charge inside the soma exceeds a certain threshold, an electric current is transmitted through the axon. "But why?," you may be wondering.

We have already commented how, when receptors get stimulated by molecules that bind to them, they can lead to the opening or closing of channels. If the effect these stimulated receptors have over the channels leads to an increase in the amount of positive charge inside the neuron's soma then the firing of an action potential will be facilitated, whereas if the change triggered by the stimulated receptor leads to a reduction in the overall positive charge inside the neuron's soma, the neuron will be

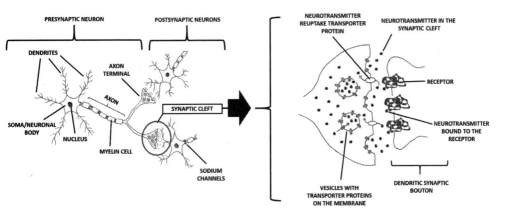

Figure 3. A presynaptic neuron and two postsynaptic neurons are shown on the *left.* Dendrites and an axon with sodium channels, surrounded by flat cells forming the insulating myelin sheath, can be seen emerging from the soma. On the *right,* the synaptic cleft is shown in more detail. The vesicles contain proteins in their membrane that allow the neurotransmitter to enter it, and the reuptake proteins in the axon terminal's membrane reintroduce the neurotransmitter from the synaptic cleft, back into the presynaptic neuron. The synaptic bouton of the dendrites, where the receptors are located, can also be seen.

inhibited and unable to fire an action potential.[8] This is because, located at the beginning of the axon, and all along it, lie specific voltage-sensitive channels, which change conformation when the positive charge inside the neuron reaches a certain threshold. More specifically, when this threshold is reached, the channels change shape in such a way that they create a pore in the axonal membrane. These voltage-gated channels are selective to sodium (which is positively charged) and because the interior of the neuron is more negative than the exterior, when these voltage-dependent sodium channels open, more sodium enters the cell. This in turn triggers the opening of the next voltage-dependent sodium channel located along the axonal membrane, which subsequently opens up the next channel, and the next and the next, until the increases in positive charge reach the axon

8. When the difference in charge between the inside and the outside of a cell becomes smaller, we say that the cell gets depolarized (the positive-negative pole present across the membrane is reduced), and when it becomes bigger, we say it becomes hyperpolarized.

Scan the QR code to see a short animation of an action potential propagated along the axon. GIF by Laurentaylorj.

terminal.[9] Through this fancy mechanism, these voltage-sensitive channels allow the action potential to propagate throughout the axon until it reaches the axon terminal where it signals the release of neurotransmitters. The propagation of the action potential along the axon is well exemplified in the GIF embedded inside the QR code above.

The sodium channels located in the axon eventually close, and there is a refractory period during which they cannot reopen, making propagation unidirectional. And, although on some occasions the electrical current may, for reasons we will not go into here, propagate from the axon terminal to the neuronal soma, most electrical currents propagate from the neuronal soma to the axon terminal, which signals the release of neurotransmitters.

Once the neuron has generated an action potential it must return to its resting state (in which the interior is more negative than the exterior) in order to be able to generate new action potentials. This is accomplished through other membrane-localized proteins called sodium-potassium pumps, which, using energy, move ions across the membrane against their electrochemical gradient, bringing the internal state of the neuron to a state where it can once again become depolarized and fire another action potential.

Whether or not the internal positive charge exceeds the threshold that opens up the sodium channels depends on the totality of signals that

---

9. Molecules that promote depolarization are excitatory and facilitate the firing of action potentials whereas molecules that promote hyperpolarization are inhibitory and reduce the likelihood of the neuron firing an action potential.

are reaching the neuron's dendrites at any given moment, each synapse contributing to the total balance of charges within the neuron. In this way, and to reduce the likelihood of the neuron spontaneously firing an action potential, the threshold is usually exceeded only when the neuron receives several signals simultaneously, capable of transferring the increase in positive charge through the entire neuronal soma until it reaches the beginning of the axon. Each synapse contributes to this balance, so the neuron, therefore, functions as a coincidence detector, firing an action potential only when a series of signals coincides. Furthermore, depending on what the neuron detects, synapses can be strengthened or weakened, giving the nervous system a great deal of plasticity (we will study in more detail how this neuroplasticity occurs in the next section).

In short, this is how a neuron works. Depending on whether or not there is enough positive charge in the neuron's soma, which in turn depends, among other things, on the signals detected by the receptors, an action potential will be generated or not. If this happens, the neuron will release a neurotransmitter, and if the next neuron receives enough excitatory signals, it will also generate an action potential, thus transferring the information through the nervous system.

Neuroplasticity

Neuroplasticity refers to the brain's ability to form and reorganize synaptic connections, especially in response to learning, new experiences, or following injury.

As we will see further on, the neurotransmitter released by cortical neurons is mainly glutamate, and it plays a fundamental role in establishing the synaptic strengths between neurons. Glutamate carries out this synaptic reinforcement through two of its receptors: the amino-3-hydroxy-5-methyl-4-isoxazole propionic acid (AMPA) and the N-methyl-D-aspartate (NMDA) receptors. Both glutamatergic receptors have an excitatory effect on the neuron (i.e., they increase the positive charge inside the cell) and, behaving in very different ways, work together to modify synaptic strengths, both to weaken or strengthen the synapse.

Both AMPA and NMDA receptors form a pore in the membrane, but in the NMDA receptor this pore is blocked by a positively charged magnesium ion, which glutamate-binding alone cannot remove. Hence, this receptor will not be able to exert its action over the neuron until this ion is removed from here, something that is only achieved when very high levels of positive charge, capable of repelling this positive ion, are reached inside the neuron (step 4 in figure 4). Only then will the channel be free and the NMDA receptor activated.

In contrast, glutamate does activate the AMPA receptor directly and, when it does, the AMPA receptor begins to allow sodium (Na+) to enter the neuron (step 2 in figure 4). When the concentration of glutamate outside the neuron causes an intense and frequent activation of AMPA receptors that is strong enough to generate an action potential,

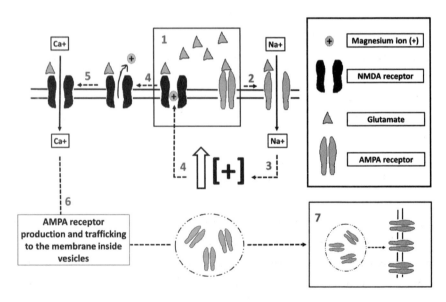

Figure 4. Mechanism of neuroplasticity through which a glutamatergic synapse in the cortex is strengthened. Step 1, glutamate binds to NMDA receptor and AMPA; step 2, activation of AMPA; step 3, increase in positive charge inside the neuron through AMPA; step 4, positive charge in the interior of the neuron reaches a threshold that repels the magnesium ion unblocking the NMDA receptor; step 5, massive calcium influx; step 6, intracellular signaling; and step 7, insertion of AMPA receptors into the membrane. (See also color plate 1.)

the levels of positive charge inside the neuron will exceed the threshold required to repel the magnesium ion that blocks the NDMA receptor (step 4 in figure 4). Once this happens, a massive influx of calcium will enter the neuron via the NDMA receptor (step 5 in figure 4), signaling the need to produce and incorporate more AMPA receptors into the synaptic bouton (steps 6 and 7 in figure 4). This increase in AMPA receptors on the postsynaptic neuron's membrane, in turn, increases the number of pores through which the positive charge can enter the neuron, the end result being that, for the same amount of glutamate in the synaptic cleft as before the AMPA reinforcement, the neuron is now capable of generating an action potential faster.

In conclusion, through this mechanism, the neuron detects whether there is a reliable and significant input of information, and once detected, by increasing the number of AMPA receptors in the membrane, it increases the strength of the synapses involved in the transmission of this information, making it easier for the postsynaptic neuron to trigger an action potential and, more efficiently, transmit the information to the next levels. Incredible cell adaptation and cooperation between different proteins in the cell membrane!

Neuroplasticity is not just about strengthening or weakening synapses. Until recently, the regenerative capacity of the adult brain was thought to be nonexistent because, unlike most tissues, the neurons that make up the nervous tissue are not replaced throughout life. This led to the belief that, once adulthood was reached, the birth of new neurons was impossible. However, in the last twenty years, three areas of the brain have been discovered where stem cells reside, i.e., pluripotent cells that can transform into neurons when they receive certain signals. One of these is an area of the hippocampus, another an area of the amygdala, and the third is an area of the prefrontal cortex (we will study these areas in detail later), and this birth or proliferation of new neurons is called neurogenesis. In addition, neuroplasticity also consists in the formation of new synaptic boutons (synaptogenesis) as well as in the growth of new dendrites and axons (neuritogenesis). In chapter 4, we will see how psychedelics seem to promote all these processes!

Neurotransmitters and Receptors:
A Complex World

Generally, neurons synthesize only one type of neurotransmitter, and these are synthesized in different areas of the nervous system. For example, neurotransmitters belonging to the monoamine family (dopamine, serotonin, and noradrenaline) are synthesized almost exclusively in very specific subcortical areas. Dopamine, involved in motivation, cognition, and movement, is synthesized only in subcortical areas known as the substantia nigra and the ventral tegmental area. Serotonin, involved in the regulation of sleep, anxiety, and mood, is only synthesized in neurons located in a cluster of nuclei, the raphe nuclei, found in the brain stem (although curiously it is also synthesized heavily outside the nervous system, specifically in the digestive tract). And noradrenaline, which is involved in monitoring the environment and maintaining appropriate levels of alertness, is synthesized in neurons in another nucleus of the brain stem called the locus coeruleus[10] (it is also synthesized outside of the nervous system, for example, in the kidney's adrenal gland, where it acts as a hormone).

Neurons located in each of these subcortical nuclei send long projections to the cortex, flooding it with their respective neurotransmitters. Figure 5, for example, shows the serotonergic projections. As you can see, these leave the raphe nuclei and flood the cortex with serotonin.

Other neurotransmitters such as glutamate or gamma-aminobutyric acid, known as GABA, are synthesized by cortical neurons, with only one-fifth of these neurons being GABAergic (i.e., synthesizing GABA) and the remainder glutamatergic (i.e., synthesizing glutamate). GABA is the inhibitory neurotransmitter par excellence in the nervous system and this inhibitory function plays

---

10. The functions presented here for each of these neurotransmitters are greatly simplified as the same function requires a combination of multiple neurotransmitters. These also interact with each other to carry out the functions described, and there is a multitude of different receptors for each neurotransmitter, these being what ultimately determines the action that the neurotransmitter will have on the nervous system.

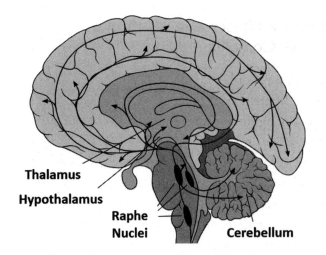

Thalamus

Hypothalamus

Raphe Nuclei

Cerebellum

Figure 5. Serotonergic projections leaving the raphe nuclei located in the brain stem. Image by Patrick J. Lynch, medical illustrator.

a fundamental role in regulating the activity of neuronal circuits. For example, a glutamatergic neuron (neuron A) may be inhibited by an inhibitory neuron (neuron B) and, to activate neuron A, another inhibitory neuron (neuron C) will need to inhibit neuron B. Unlike GABA, glutamate is the excitatory neurotransmitter synthesized by the cortex, although as we will see when we delve into psychedelic neuroscience, this is not so straightforward, because some glutamate receptors can also exert an inhibitory action.

As it has become clear so far, the complexity of the nervous system is not only limited to the different neurotransmitters[11] but instead lies largely in their interaction with different receptors. There are, for example, five families of receptors to which serotonin can bind, and within each of these families, there are in turn several subtypes, each with a molecular conformation, a distribution map, and a specific effect on the neuron. As if this were not enough, and as we will see when we study the action of psychedelic molecules, the cascade of information unleashed by each of these receptors can vary depending on the specific molecule with which it is interacting at any given moment. And you should know that receptors also interact with other receptors!

11. There are many more neurotransmitters in the nervous system than those presented here.

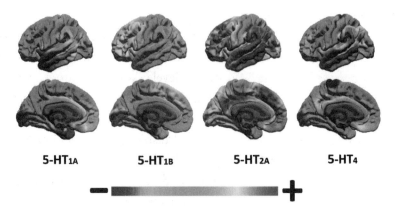

5-HT₁ₐ   5-HT₁ᵦ   5-HT₂ₐ   5-HT₄

Figure 6. Distribution maps of four types of serotonin (5-HT) receptors: two from family 1, one from family 2, and one from family 4. The areas with a high density of the corresponding receptor and the areas with a lower density can be seen. Image obtained from a study led by Beliveau et al. (2017). (See also color plate 2.)

Finally, consider that, in a given neuron, there are many different receptors. In figure 6[12] you can see the distribution maps of some serotonin receptors. Note that there are notable differences between maps, as well as a clear overlap between them in certain areas.

Imagine the unfathomable complexity of the nervous system when you consider that there are billions of neurons in it and that the final state of each one of them depends on the combination of neurotransmitters being detected by a multitude of different receptors at thousands of synapses distributed across the neuronal membrane, each one of them contributing to the final behavior of the neuron! Mind boggling!

A Rich Consciousness: Senses, Thalamus, and Cerebral Cortex

After traveling inside the complex world of a neuron, it is time to zoom out and look at the nervous system as a whole in order to visualize how it integrates all the information into a rich conscious experience.

---

12. Beliveau V, Ganz M, Feng L, Ozenne B, Højgaard L, Fisher PM, Knudsen GM. 2017. A high-resolution in vivo atlas of the human brain's serotonin system. Journal of Neuroscience 37(1):120–128.

Integrating Information

For integration to occur, it is essential that information from neurons at the first level, or first-order neurons, converges in an orderly and segregated fashion on neurons at higher levels. When a neuron from the second level then fires an action potential, it will contain an integrated version of all the information contained in the lower-order neurons that have converged on it. In a hierarchical fashion, the second-order neurons will send the information to the third-order ones and so on. Thus, at each step, a more and more integrated version of the external information is formed until culminating in a conscious experience. You can see a representation of this process in figure 7.

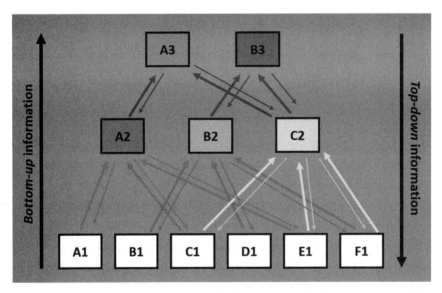

Figure 7. Diagram of the convergence of information. In this diagram, neuron A2, placed at the second level of integration is receiving information from the first-order neurons A1, C1, and E1, while the second-order neuron B2 is receiving information from the first-order neurons B1, D1, and F1. Equally, neuron C2 is receiving information from C1, E1, and F1. When neuron A2 fires an action potential to the corresponding third-order neuron (A3), it will transmit integrated information from A1, C1, and E1, while neuron B2 will transmit integrated information from B1, D1, and F1. And in the same way, information from second-order neurons will converge on third-order ones. Regulatory information (i.e., top-down information from higher to lower levels) is also shown. (See also color plate 3.)

This is, of course, an extremely simplified version that helps us get an idea of how information that is initially segregated becomes organized and integrated through hierarchical levels to finally give rise to a unitary experience. In addition to these bottom-up projections that send information from lower levels to higher levels, connections between neurons at the same level also exist, as do top-down projections that go from higher to lower levels. As will be explained further on, these top-down projections represent a key component, since by involving inhibitory processes, they regulate what information from lower levels reaches higher ones.

From the Senses to the Cortex: Reentrant Cortico-Thalamic Projections

How do we become conscious of the information picked up by the senses? To answer this question, we have to look at the trajectory that the sensory information follows, from the moment when we are first exposed to it until it becomes part of our conscious experience. Logically, this process begins in our sensory organs, whose neurons have specific receptors in their membranes through which they are capable of interacting with different stimuli from the outside world. For example, neurons in the first layer of the eye's retina have a photosensitive protein called rhodopsin. That is, it interacts with the electromagnetic waves generated by photons and in doing so, changes its conformation, causing the neuron to release the neurotransmitter to the next layer of neurons in the retina, which in turn pass the information to the next layer.

In the inner ear, the auditory sensory cells have tiny "hairs" called cilia. The mechanical forces within sound waves move them, initiating a signal that culminates in the release of a neurotransmitter to the next neuron. Receptors in the skin also respond to mechanical force, while receptors in taste buds and olfactory neurons detect molecules through chemically interacting with them.

The final destination of the information originating in the sensory organs is the cerebral cortex, which is the outermost structure of the brain. This structure is divided into two hemispheres, each consisting of five lobes: occipital, temporal, parietal, frontal, and limbic (figure 8). The first three are sensorial: the occipital lobe receives visual informa-

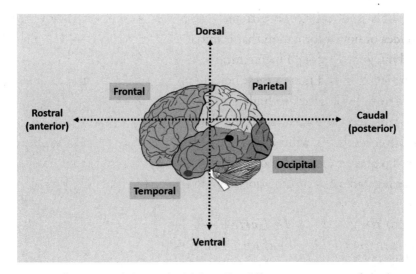

Figure 8. Illustration of the cerebral lobes. The different orientations of the brain are also shown, which apply to all brain lobes (e.g., the gray dot is located in the anteroventral temporal lobe and the black dot in the posterodorsal temporal lobe). (See also color plate 4.)

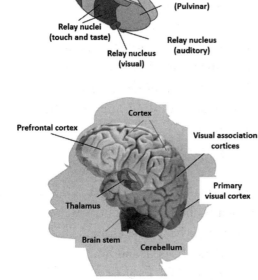

Figure 9. A schematic representation of some thalamic nuclei (*above*) and their corresponding cortical projections (*below*). Image by Nadal and Amarillo (2018). (See also color plate 5.)

tion, the temporal one auditory, and the parietal one somatosensory information (i.e., information from the tongue and skin). The frontal lobe is responsible for selecting and executing the actions required to meet the individual's goals, which will depend on their inner drive and on the stimuli present in the environment (and in humans, also on abstract representations).

Except for olfactory information, which travels directly from the olfactory bulb to the olfactory cortex, all other information coming in through our senses is first transmitted to the thalamus, a key structure located in the center of the brain. The thalamus is not a homogeneous structure; it is made up of many different nuclei of neurons, defined according to what information they receive and where they send it to, and they are highly connected to the cortex. Not only do they send projections there (i.e., thalamocortical projections), but they also receive a multitude of direct projections from it (i.e., corticothalamic projections). Within the corticothalamic projections, we can find reciprocal ones, which travel back to the same thalamic nuclei from which the cortical neurons were receiving information, and nonreciprocal ones, which send information to a different, higher-order, thalamic nucleus.

Sensory information arrives separately at the thalamus, meaning that each sensory organ sends information to its corresponding thalamic nucleus (red arrows in color plate 6), which is unimodal (i.e., it

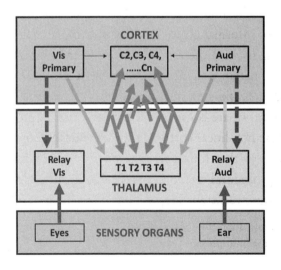

Figure 10. The box at the *bottom* represents the sensory organs. The box in the *middle* represents the thalamus and the box *above* the cortex. T1, T2, T3, T4: association thalamic nuclei; C2, C3, C4 ... Cn: heteromodal and associative cortices; Aud: auditory; Vis: visual. (See also color plate 6.)

receives only one type of sensory information). These unimodal nuclei are called sensory thalamic relay nuclei because they pass, or relay, that information to their corresponding sensory cortex (yellow arrows in color plate 6), namely, to the primary sensory cortex (i.e., the first-order cortical areas where sensory information that has not yet been processed by the cortex arrives). In addition to these sensory relay nuclei, there is also a motor relay nucleus. This nucleus indirectly, and via a subcortical structure discussed later (the striatum), receives information from the motor association cortex and controls the activation of the primary motor cortex, the latter in charge of sending projections to the spinal cord where it activates neurons directly in charge of activating the muscles (i.e., motor neurons). Moreover, there is also a limbic relay nucleus, but we will focus on it when studying the limbic system.

Once the sensory information reaches the primary cortex, it is sent back to the thalamus through the corticothalamic projections. As we mentioned above, some of it goes back to the thalamic relay nucleus, but some is sent to higher-order thalamic nuclei, namely, the thalamic association nuclei. There, visual information, for example, converges with limbic or auditory information (green arrows in color plate 6), as well as with information from other thalamic nuclei. These association nuclei now send projections to heteromodal and associative cortical areas,[13] which in turn send projections back to other thalamic nuclei, and these, once again, send projections back to the cortex. This way, reentrant projections are formed between the thalamus and the cortex, allowing a deep and progressive integration of information to occur (blue arrows in color plate 6) capable of providing us with the richness found in the human, and more generally, the mammalian, conscious experience. In *A Universe of Consciousness: How Matter Becomes Imagination*, Gerald M. Edelman and Giulio Tononi argue that we are conscious of the information processed through precisely these non-linear corticothalamic reentrant loops, comparing this architecture to that found in systems involved in the processing of unconscious procedural memory, which, unlike the architecture of the cortico-thalamic reentrant loops, depends on linear and

---

13. Heteromodal areas process information from various senses, while associative areas also include motor, limbic, and verbal information.

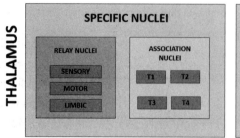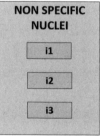

Figure 11. Schematic representation of the thalamic nuclei.

unidirectional pathways formed between the cerebellum, the basal ganglia, the thalamus, and the cortex.

The relay and association thalamic nuclei have very well-defined projections, but the thalamus also contains dispersed groups of neurons forming the nonspecific thalamic nuclei. Unlike the relay and association ones, the nonspecific thalamic nuclei send diffuse projections to both the brain and other thalamic nuclei and play a key role in synchronizing the activity of the different brain regions. Figure 11 shows a schematic representation of these thalamic nuclei.

Regulation of Thalamic Activity

Two main mechanisms exist through which thalamic activity is regulated. One is through the thalamic reticular nucleus (a nonspecific nucleus), and the other is through the striatum (a set of subcortical inhibitory structures). In chapter 4, we will see how psychedelics possibly affect both of these regulatory mechanisms.

Thalamic Reticular Nucleus

The thalamic reticular nucleus (TRN) surrounds the main body of the thalamus (where the specific nuclei sit) and is positioned between it and the cortex. As they leave the thalamus, the thalamocortical projections send collaterals to the neurons from this nucleus, informing them of the information they are carrying to the cortex. The reciprocal corticothalamic projections (i.e., those that go to the same thalamic nucleus from which they receive information) also send collaterals here (figure 12).

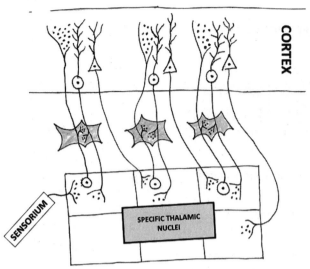

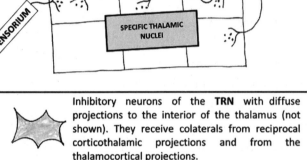

Inhibitory neurons of the **TRN** with diffuse projections to the interior of the thalamus (not shown). They receive colaterals from reciprocal corticothalamic projections and from the thalamocortical projections.

Figure 12. The figure shows neurons from the thalamic reticular nucleus (TRN) positioned between the specific thalamic nuclei and the cortex. For simplicity, the diffuse inhibitory projections leaving the TRN toward the main body of the thalamus are not shown.

This nonspecific nucleus is composed solely of inhibitory neurons and these simultaneously send diffuse projections to several specific thalamic nuclei (not shown in figure 12). This endows this nucleus with the ability to finely coordinate the upstream of thalamic information to the cortex. For example, when we sleep, neurons in this nucleus begin to fire rhythmically, which prevents the sensory information from ascending to the cortex and waking us up.

The Striatum

Thalamic activity is also regulated via the striatum, a set of inhibitory subcortical structures. GABAergic neurons in one of these structures (known as the internal pallidum) send inhibitory projections to the thalamic nuclei, thereby controlling their activity and, consequently, the activity of the cortical area into which the thalamic nucleus in question projects, but what determines whether the neurons of the internal pallidum are inhibiting the thalamus or not? How is the state

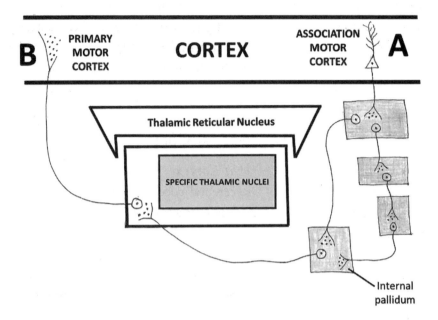

Figure 13. Schematic representation of a cortico-striatal-thalamo-cortical loop starting in cortical area A and controlling cortical area B. The motor loop is shown as an example, but there are others. The striatum is represented by the set of four shaded squares on the *right*. These subcortical structures are made up of inhibitory neurons that form various circuits through which they control the activity of the internal pallidum and, consequently, the inhibition/activation of the thalamic nuclei.

of this inhibitory structure controlled? This is where the other structures of the striatum come into play since these form various circuits through which they manage to inhibit the internal pallidum, thus releasing the brake that was halting the thalamic information from reaching the cortex. In other words, some parts of the striatum (the internal pallidum) inhibit the thalamic nuclei and other parts inhibit the inhibitor.[14] We will not study these striatal circuits in more detail. All you need to know is that these structures are controlled by neurons in the deep layers of the cortex and that they form part of important

---

14. This dance between activation and inhibition within both serial and circular circuits is an extremely prevalent and elegant regulatory mechanism found not only in neuronal circuits, but at the level of the molecular reactions occurring inside single cells. For example, many enzymes are inhibited by the product of the reaction they catalyze.

cortico-striatal-thalamocortical loops. Through these loops, a particular area of the cortex (area A in figure 13) can control the activity of another distal cortical area (area B in figure 13) by regulating the effect that the striatum has on the thalamic nucleus that projects to area B in the diagram.

The Cerebral Cortex

Neuroanatomy of the Cerebral Cortex

It is now time to focus on the cerebral cortex and study its anatomy in more detail. We know of no other structure in the universe of such complexity!

In addition to sending projections to subcortical structures such as the thalamus or the striatum, the neurons in the cortex also communicate horizontally among them. We will refer to the projections from the cortex to the subcortical structures as vertical projections and to cortico-cortical projections as horizontal ones. Thus, this structure is organized both horizontally and vertically, as you can see in figure 14.

Horizontally, the cortex is made up of several layers. These layers are differentiated according to the type of neurons that reside within them; where they receive their inputs from and where they send their outputs to. Neurons located in the most *superficial layers* do not send vertical projections to the thalamus but instead send horizontal projections to other areas of the cortex. For the most part, they transmit information from the lower levels of integration to the higher levels. This information ascends and is thus called *bottom-up information*. In figure 14, these bottom-up horizontal projections are indicated by the arrows pointing to the right.

Meanwhile, as represented by the arrows pointing to the left in figure 14, deep layers send horizontal information mostly in the opposite direction: from higher levels to lower ones in what is termed top-down information, which using inhibitory processes, regulates the bottom-up information, as we will see in more detail in the section of this chapter called "Theory of Hierarchical Predictive Coding."

So far, we have studied how the cerebral cortex is organized horizontally into layers of differentiated cells. Now, let's study its horizontal architecture.

The dendrites of the deep cortical neurons are long and extent upwards, reaching the superficial layers of the cortex,[15] collecting a multitude of information from there. Furthermore, in addition to the top-down horizontal projections, the neurons in the deep layers of the cortex also send vertical projections to subthalamic nuclei (the arrows pointing downward in figure 14), not only to higher-order thalamic nuclei, but also to the same thalamic nucleus from which they receive information from, regulating it (i.e., dashed-purple arrows in color plate 6 showing reciprocal regulatory projections).

Thanks to these neuroanatomical characteristics, the cortex is also organized into vertical functional units called cortical columns, with each cortical column representing a particular order of integration. Figure 14 shows three of these vertical units. Within each column exist closed neuronal circuits formed by neurons of the same cortical column located at different heights. Due to the inherent complexity of these circuits, they are not shown in figure 14, but they integrate information from adjacent columns, from both lower- and higher-order ones, as well as information from the thalamus, carrying out complex computations and sending the result both horizontally to other adjacent columns and vertically to subcortical structures.

In addition to the vertical corticothalamic projections, we have already mentioned that vertical projections to the striatum also exist and that these indirectly regulate thalamic activity and thus the activity of the cortex itself (figure 13).

Finally, we must remember that the majority (80 percent) of neurons in the cortex are glutamatergic. That is, they receive information from a multitude of neurotransmitters released by neurons in the subcortical nuclei (e.g., serotonergic raphe nuclei), but respond only by releasing glutamate. The remaining 20 percent of cortical neurons are inhibitory neurons. That is, they respond by releasing the neurotransmitter

---

15. A neuron's body can have dendritic extensions in many different directions. The dendrites that go upward are called apical dendrites.

THREE COLUMNS OF THE CEREBRAL CORTEX

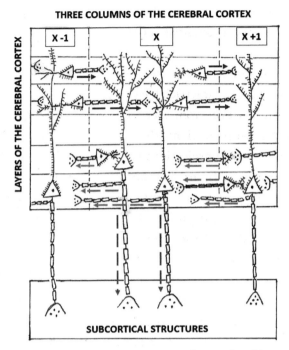

Figure 14. Simplified schematic representation of vertical and horizontal cortical projections. The figure shows three cortical columns of ascending levels of integration (X-1, X, and X+1) and six horizontal layers. Each triangle represents the neuronal body from which dendrites (represented by the thin lines) and axons (represented with the myelin sheaths) emerge. The neurotransmitters released by the axon terminals are represented by the black dots. The arrows represent the three different types of projections. There are two types of horizontal projections: bottom-up projections, which go from lower- to higher-order columns, are represented by the arrows pointing to the right; and top-down projections, which go from the higher- to the lower-order columns, are represented by the arrows pointing to the left. The vertical projections that send information from the deep cortical layers to subcortical structures are represented by the arrows pointing downward.

GABA. Within the cortex, glutamatergic neurons have long projections, whereas GABAergic neurons are small neurons that act locally by regulating the activity of cortical neurons. This type of small and local neuron is referred to as an interneuron. In contrast to these cortical interneurons, inhibitory neurons in the striatum send long inhibitory projections to other nuclei in the striatum, as well as to the thalamus.

In short, by now you will have noticed that the integration process that allows conscious experience does not only depend on information converging in an orderly fashion at higher and higher-order levels through the re-entrant projections between the thalamus and the cortex (i.e., bottom-up information) but that the inhibitory mechanisms (i.e., top-down information) through which the different brain structures regulate the information that the lower levels project onto them are also fundamental. We have also seen two mechanisms of thalamic regulation through which the cortex, in turn, regulates itself:

1. The reciprocal corticothalamic projections that enable cortical autoregulation through the thalamic reticular nucleus shown in the lower image of figure 12.
2. The cortico-striatal-thalamo-cortical loops shown in figure 13.

Theory of Hierarchical Predictive Coding

According to the theory of hierarchical predictive coding, as the brain receives information throughout life, it stores it in the form of a functionally summarized model of the world. This model is then used to make predictions about the causes of stimuli and the consequences of actions. What we perceive at any given moment is not reality, but the model we have constructed, which, according to this theory, is constantly being compared with incoming information (i.e., bottom-up information). When it detects that the incoming information does not coincide with the model (i.e., top-down information), it generates a signal called a "prediction error," which contains the new information and is sent to higher-order levels and used to update the models contained there. If the brain instead detects that the incoming information is already included in the model, there will be no need to send this incoming information to higher orders and its ascent will be suppressed by the top-down inhibitory projections.

How does the brain, according to this theory, carry out these calculations? This theory encompasses a multitude of formulas and it is of great complexity, but I will explain it as best as I can. Be aware that the explanation below is highly simplified.

Having said this, let's return to the organization of the cerebral cortex. Recall that, through its most superficial layers, each cortical column sends cortico-cortical information mostly to higher-order columns (i.e., ascending/bottom-up horizontal projections), and through its deep layers, sends mostly cortico-cortical projections to the lower-order columns (i.e., descending/top-down horizontal projections), as well as projections to the thalamus (i.e., vertical projections). In an extremely simplified form, what the theory of hierarchical predictive coding postulates is that by comparing the information from the deep layers with that from the superficial layers, and taking into consideration the thalamic inputs too, the circuit within each column calculates a prediction error (figure 15[16]).

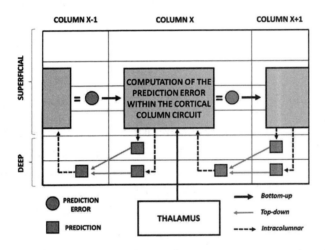

Figure 15. This figure shows three columns of successive integration orders: (X-1), (X), and (X+1). In the closed circuit within each column, a prediction error is calculated taking into consideration: 1) the prediction/expectation of the higher-order column (i.e., top-down information); 2) the bottom-up information of the adjacent lower-order column transferring its own prediction error; and 3) the bottom-up information of the thalamus. Note that the prediction error calculated in each column represents the bottom-up information sent to the next column. The black arrows represent bottom-up information, the gray arrows top-down information, and the dotted arrows, intracolumn information. Image modified from Shipp (2016).

---

16. Simplified image from the following article: Shipp S. 2016. Neural elements for predictive coding. Frontiers in Psychology 7:1792.

This prediction error becomes the bottom-up information that this column (i.e., X–1) will send through its superficial layers to the next higher-order column (i.e., X). In this next column (i.e., X), this incoming bottom-up information will be compared with the top-down information carrying the prediction received from the deep layers of the next higher-order column (i.e., X+1). This way, column X will calculate its own prediction error which it will send, through its superficial layers, to the next higher-order column X+1. In an attempt to reduce the prediction errors within the system, each column will use the prediction errors it receives to update the predictions it sends down to its associated lower-order column. Prediction errors will step up the integration hierarchy until either the prediction of a higher level contains the information conveyed in it, in which case such prediction will prevent the prediction error from stepping up further, or until it reaches the top of the integration hierarchy.

Let's reflect upon the fact that prediction errors are transmitted through the action potentials generated by neurons in the superficial layers and signal the need to introduce new information into the model of the world (i.e., modify the synaptic strength map of the brain). If the prediction error arriving at column X is already contained in the prediction of column X+1, the generation of the action potential that would incorporate that information into the model will be inhibited. After all, the model already includes that information! In short, according to this theory, prediction errors represent bottom-up cortical information, and the predictions made by the model represent cortical top-down information.

Finally, we should mention that each prediction error and each expectation/prediction are associated with a certain precision. That is, how much can I rely on the bottom-up and on top-down information at each level when calculating a prediction error? The precision associated with each one of these will determine the final result.

A very classic example used to understand this notion is the Charles Bonnet syndrome in which elderly people who have lost visual capacity start to have visual hallucinations. According to predictive coding theory, this occurs because the loss of vision makes incoming information very "noisy" and full of artefacts. In other words, the bottom-up information loses precision. When calculating the prediction error, the cortical column will take into account the low accuracy associated with that incoming information, and, as the precision of the model's prediction (formed through life experience) is higher than the precision of the incoming information, the prediction of the model will dominate the experience and cause a hallucination.

Similarly, imagine, for example, that you are attracted to someone and that this person is also attracted to you but that, due to low self-esteem as a product of certain life experiences, you do not believe this is the case. Let's now imagine that this person often invites you out for a walk. Faced with this ambiguous incoming information where the precision of the incoming information is not excessively high (a walk is not a kiss!), the time it takes you to realize that your prediction is wrong (i.e. the time it takes you to update your model), will depend on the precision with which you hold such a prediction (i.e., the belief that it is unlikely that the other person likes you). If that belief has a very high associated precision, you will only be able to update the model when the incoming information has a much higher precision than that contained in the ambiguous walk. If the person, for example, finally kisses you, the precision of the incoming information related to how the person feels about you will increase, and by increasing its precision, a prediction error that was before absent will now be generated, forcing you to change the precision associated with your prediction, or even changing that prediction altogether as you now become aware that they do in fact like you back.

Hence, the prediction error calculated in column X will be the result of comparing the bottom-up information sent by column X–1 and the top-down information sent by column X+1, while additionally taking into account the precision associated with both types of information. In chapter 4 we will see how, according to this theory, psychedelics act by affecting prediction errors, predictions, and their associated precisions.

Expansion of the Association Cortex
As we saw before, the different sensory inputs originally reach different regions of the cortex termed the primary sensory regions (e.g., primary visual area, or primary auditory area). These areas only process one

type of sensory information and are thus called unimodal areas. The information from these unimodal areas then converges in higher-order regions of the cortex called the heteromodal cortices, involved in processing and integrating sensory inputs from different modalities. Lastly, this highly integrated sensory information is integrated further with motor and emotional information in the association cortices.

The number of computations carried out when integrating the information picked up by the different senses has been increasing throughout evolution. This is clearly seen in figure 16,[17] which shows how the association cortices located between the primary areas have been undoubtedly expanding over time.

Imagine all the visual perceptions that have existed of the same photon (i.e., light particle). The experience that a dog has from a particular photon will be very different from that of a human being, or from that of an ant or a bird. Each organism will generate a unique integrated representation of such a stimulus, not to mention all the other sensory organs present in nature beyond those found in humans! Fish perceive electric fields and snakes perceive thermodynamic ones, to give just a couple of examples.

Isn't it fascinating? The universe developing infinite ways of exploring itself, infinite ways of integrating all the information that, for some as yet unknown reason is "out there," patiently waiting for a system to develop with receptors capable of capturing it and complex mechanisms capable of integrating it.

The Prefrontal Cortex

As can be seen in figure 9 and figure 17, the prefrontal cortex (PFC) occupies a large part of the frontal lobe. It represents the most recent phylogenetic and associative areas of this motor lobe, and here converges highly integrated information from the outside world with information from the internal world (i.e., from memory and the body) needed to decide what actions the individual should perform.

---

17. Image obtained from the following article: Buckner RL, Krienen FM. 2013. The evolution of distributed association networks in the human brain. Trends in Cognitive Sciences 17(12):648–665.

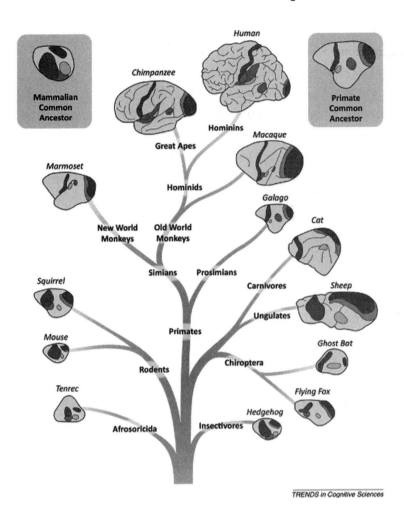

Figure 16. Phylogenetic tree of the brain. The shaded areas show the different primary cortices, whereas the association cortices are shown in light gray. Image obtained from Buckner and Krienen (2013). (See also color plate 7.)

The prefrontal cortex can be divided into many different areas. And there is not just one single classification of these subdivisions in the literature but many, which is a real pain in the neck when trying to compare results obtained from different studies that do not use the same one. Nevertheless, we can broadly divide the prefrontal cortex into lateral, medial, and ventral parts. Figure 17 shows the location of these subdivisions.

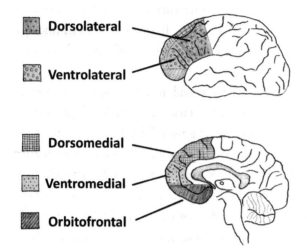

Figure 17. Subdivisions of the prefrontal cortex. A lateral plane of the brain is shown *above* and a medial plane *below*. (See also color plate 8.)

Generally speaking, the lateral parts are responsible for processing information from the outside world and are involved in processes that require high attentional control. The medial areas, instead, receive information about the individual's internal world (e.g., an imagined mental scene or conversation, the state of the body, etc.) originated in subcortical structures that we will study in the next section (the hippocampus, the amygdala, and the insula). As we will see toward the end of the chapter, these medial prefrontal areas are highly active when, without making an active effort to control attention, our mind wanders. And they are also highly active when we activate the representation of one's self.

The division between medial and lateral areas does not apply to the most ventral area of the prefrontal cortex, located just above the eyes and known as the orbitofrontal cortex. As we will see shortly, the hippocampus (a structure highly involved in memory and in building mental scenes) projects extensively to this area.

The Limbic System

After studying how perceptual processes work and how the brain integrates information and builds a model of the world, we must focus on yet another component that always accompanies us: emotions. This component is essential, since it is the one that guides us humans (and other animals too) in our decision making. It is the brain's limbic system, which consists of a set of areas involved in judgmental, motivational, and decision-making processes.

That which is necessary for our survival and development causes us pleasure, and that which is threatening causes us pain. Look at how far evolution has come with this simple mechanism. This is already present in some bacteria that, when sensing sugar in their environment, move toward it and when sensing acid, move away. Based on this simple principle, evolution has gradually developed the complex behavior of human beings. Humans not only move closer or farther away, depending on the stimuli in their environment; they are also capable of generating representations in their minds. On the one hand, we are capable of imagining threatening situations, those that impede our development and cause us pain, suffering, and fear. This is the evaluative or judgmental part of the limbic system. On the other hand, we are also capable of imagining those things or events that we feel are necessary for our development, to *desire them*, and to plan the actions required to achieve such goals and thus, obtain pleasure and happiness. These are the motivational aspects of the limbic system.

Neuroanatomy of the Limbic System

Let's study which subcortical structures are involved in these processes. In figure 18 and figure 19 you can find the spatial location of some of the areas that we will mention below, although, given the complexity of the matter, not all of them are included.

The Hippocampus

The imaginative capacity involved in both evaluative and motivational processes depends to a large extent on our ability to use past information to construct new scenarios. The subcortical structure par excellence involved in memory encoding and reconstruction is the hippocampus. The olfactory cortex, which receives direct input from the olfactory bulb (without passing through the thalamus) projects directly to the hippocampus, which is why smells have such a strong ability to evoke memories. And memories are tightly linked to emotions.

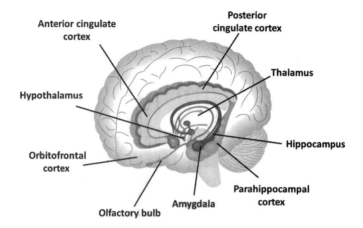

Figure 18. Location of some of the main structures of the limbic system. Image modified and obtained from DataBase Center for Life Science.

Do you remember that when we studied the relay nuclei of the thalamus, we mentioned that there was one that received information from the limbic system? Well, it is particularly from the hippocampus that this nucleus receives extensive projections. Once here, the information is sent to cortical areas involved in limbic processes. On the one hand,

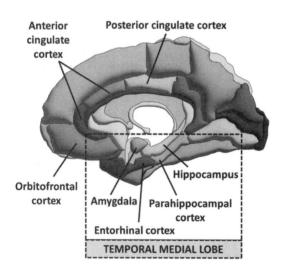

Figure 19. Visual representation of the cortical areas of the medial temporal lobe. Note their proximity to the hippocampus. (See also color plate 9.)

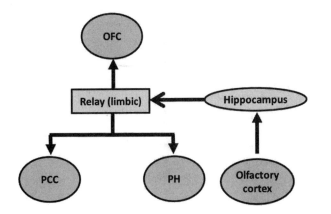

Figure 20. The hippocampus. PCC: posterior cingulate cortex, PH: parahippocampal cortex, and OFC: orbitofrontal cortex.

it projects information to the cortices surrounding the hippocampus, such as the parahippocampal cortex (PH) located in the medial part of the temporal lobe (figure 19). It also projects to the orbitofrontal cortex (OFC) and the posterior cingulate cortex (PCC) (figure 20). As we will see when we study a famous clinical case at the end of this section, the former is highly involved in impulse and emotion control and is located in the most ventral part of the frontal lobe. Regarding the PCC, this is a central node of the default mode network, an important brain network that we will study in detail toward the end of this chapter. In chapter 3 we will see how psychedelics have profound effects on the behavior of these areas.

The Amygdala

In addition to sending projections to the limbic relay nucleus of the thalamus, the hippocampus also projects extensively to another subcortical structure involved in evaluating the emotional valence of information: the amygdala. These two structures work closely together because emotionally charged events need to be encoded much more strongly than insignificant ones. Moreover, when assessing whether a stimulus is positive or negative, it is necessary to recollect previous experiences related to that stimulus in order to make a decision. Let's say, for example, that we have the option to reach a lake through two different paths, and that the last time we took one of those paths we were bitten by a snake. That experience, which activated the amygdala and had a high emotional content, will be encoded effectively and will participate in future decisions regarding which path to take.

In order to carry out this evaluative process, the amygdala receives a lot of information from the senses. On the one hand, it receives sensory information that has barely been processed, allowing these direct pathways to evaluate information from the environment quickly and unconsciously. For example, the amygdala receives auditory information directly from the auditory relay nucleus and olfactory information directly from the hippocampus. The visual relay nucleus does not send information to it, but the retina also sends a small collateral projection to a thalamic association nucleus, the pulvinar nucleus, and this one does send a direct projection to the amygdala. In addition to these semidirect sensory input pathways, the amygdala also receives more processed sensory information from the unimodal and heteromodal cortices.[18] See figure 21.

By combining all this information with information from the hippocampus, the amygdala is capable of determining whether environmental stimuli, or in the case of humans also those generated by the imagination,

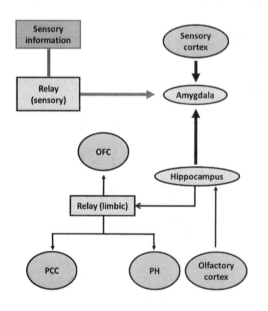

Figure 21. Inputs to the amygdala. PCC: Posterior cingulate cortex, PH: parahippocampal cortex, OFC: orbitofrontal cortex.

18. Heteromodal areas of the cortex are those where information from different sensory senses is integrated (they are not considered association areas as they are limited to processing sensory information, i.e., they don't contain motor or limbic information).

are good, bad, or indifferent to the individual. Once it has processed such information, it sends it to the rest of the system in two different ways: by projecting to the hypothalamus and to the prefrontal cortex.

Projections from the Amygdala to the Hypothalamus

The hypothalamus represents the interface between the nervous system and the endocrine (i.e., hormonal) system. When the amygdala detects any threat, it rapidly informs the hypothalamus, which is responsible for informing the autonomic nervous system (via the release of hormones) about the need to activate the appropriate physiological responses for a given moment. For example, in the face of threatening stimuli, it will activate the stress-associated release of glucocorticoids. It can also, in the face of different stimuli, release oxytocin, a hormone linked to prosocial behavior that, as we will see in chapter 5, underpins some of the effects induced by MDMA.

Inputs from the hypothalamus also reach the limbic relay nucleus of the thalamus, where it converges with inputs from the hippocampus. Thus, data regarding bodily states work together with data from memory and participate in the encoding of important information (figure 22).

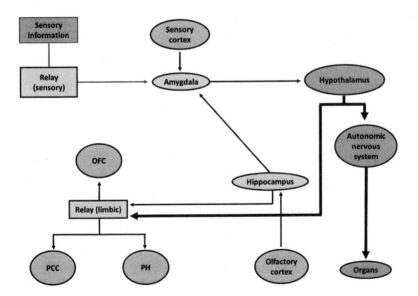

Figure 22. Output of information from the amygdala to the hypothalamus. PCC: posterior cingulate cortex, PH: parahippocampal cortex, OFC: orbitofrontal cortex.

Projections from the Amygdala to the Prefrontal Cortex
Information processed by the amygdala is sent to the prefrontal cortex where it will be used to make an informed decision about what actions to take based on current information. The amygdala projects to the prefrontal cortex both directly (to the medial prefrontal cortex) and indirectly (via the dorsomedial thalamic nucleus, an association nucleus that extensively innervates the prefrontal cortex) (figures 9 and 23).

In addition, and in a similar way to that of the thalamus, the prefrontal cortex sends a multitude of regulatory projections back to the amygdala. These activate inhibitory neurons in this subcortical structure, thus controlling its activity and playing a key role in controlling emotions (figure 23). In chapter 3, we will look at some results that suggest that the psychedelic experience is impacting this structure's ability to process negative information (at least in the safe, controlled environment in which the studies were conducted) and the implications this might have for depression.

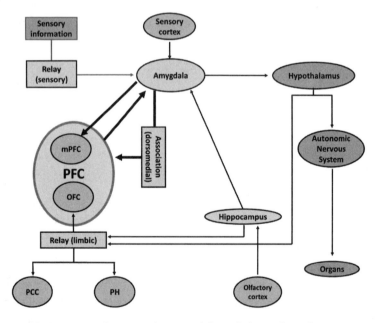

Figure 23. Projections between the amygdala and the prefrontal cortex. mPFC: medial prefrontal cortex, PCC: Posterior cingulate cortex, PFC: Prefrontal cortex, PH: Parahippocampal cortex, OFC: Orbitofrontal cortex.

The Insula

The amygdala also works closely with another complex structure: the insula. This structure is composed of both a subcortical and a cortical component (i.e., the insular cortex). In figure 24 you can see a diagram centered around this structure. It is an extremely complex structure. Through its projections to the ventromedial parts of the prefrontal cortex (vmPFC), it is involved in limbic functions, and, through its projections to the dorsal anterior cingulate cortex (ACC) and the dorsolateral prefrontal cortex (dlPFC), in cognitive ones. When, in future sections, we study how the functional architecture of the cerebral cortex is organized into brain networks, we will see how the first (i.e., vmPFC) is part of the default mode network, the second (i.e., ACC), of the ventral attentional network, and the third (i.e., dlPFC), of the frontoparietal control network; three networks that, as we will see in chapter 3, undergo profound changes during the psychedelic experience.

The amygdala and insula are highly connected, not only directly, but also through the dorsomedial thalamic nucleus (figure 24), and, like the amygdala, the insula receives information from the senses. However,

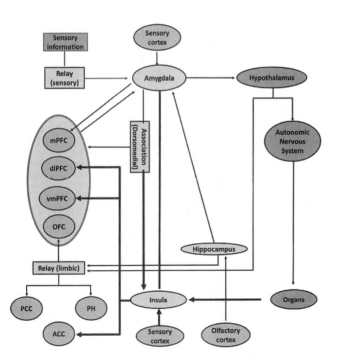

Figure 24. Input and output of information from the insula. ACC: Anterior cingulate cortex, dlPFC: dorsolateral prefrontal cortex, mPFC: medial prefrontal cortex, PCC: posterior cingulate cortex, PFC: prefrontal cortex, PH: parahippocampal cortex, OFC: orbitofrontal cortex, vmPFC: ventromedial prefrontal cortex, vmPFC: ventromedial prefrontal cortex.

unlike the amygdala, the insula also receives visceral information (i.e., information about the state of the autonomic nervous system), which, remember, was itself being modulated by the amygdala.

This makes the insula the brain structure par excellence involved in "sensing" the state of the body. As such, it is involved in the processing of physical and psychological pain, and it is also actively involved in the conscious processing of breathing, something that, as we will see throughout the book, takes prominence, both during the psychedelic experience and during meditative practices.

This structure is also highly implicated in generating a sense of agency, that is, the feeling that we humans have of being the authors (i.e., agents) behind the actions we take. This sense of agency is something we take for granted, only realizing it exists when it disappears, something that, as we shall see, occurs during the psychedelic experience.

Last but not least, the insula, as well as the limbic and cognitive cortices it projects to, plays a particularly important role in determining the personal relevance of information, which logically influences decision making. As we will see in chapter 3, psychedelics appear to promote the restructuring of the individual's relevance maps, this possibly being a major therapeutic mechanism underlying psychedelic-assisted psychotherapy. In figure 25 you can see the location of the insula and a summary of its functions.

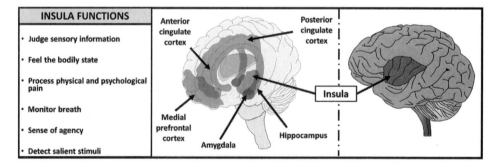

Figure 25. Functions and location of the insula. The first image shows the location of the insula in relation to the amygdala, and the second shows a more realistic representation of its location within the cortex, which is buried beneath the temporal and frontal cortex. (See also color plate 10.)

Thus, by receiving combined information from memory, the environment, and the state of the body, the prefrontal cortex is able to evaluate and make an informed judgment that will impact the decision-making process.

The Striatum

Let's now look at the motivational system, commonly known as the reward system. When a stimulus or behavior has provided a reward in the past, the animal will feel a strong motivation to repeat the behaviors that provided that reward. This motivation will instead be absent when the stimulus was insignificant or when instead of providing a reward had provided a punishment. More generally, this system is highly involved in all processes related to motor skills (e.g., motor learning and processing, initiation and regulation of voluntary movements, execution of automatic movements, and so on). The striatum is therefore actively involved in both determining what we want and what actions we need to take to achieve it.

We have already mentioned that this system is made up of a set of inhibitory subcortical structures (recall its involvement in the regulation of thalamic activity). In addition to these GABAergic structures, it also includes the substantia nigra, one of the dopaminergic nuclei of the nervous system, and also receives a strong innervation from the ventral tegmental area, another dopaminergic subcortical nucleus (figure 26).

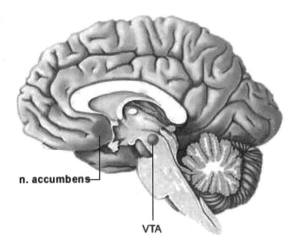

Figure 26. Medial view of the brain showing the location of the nucleus accumbens and the ventral tegmental area (VTA). Image obtained from: The brain.mcgill.ca.

This area, in particular, floods the ventral parts of the striatum with dopamine. Namely, the nucleus accumbens (figure 26). Such flooding is essential since it is the release of dopamine that drives motivated responses such as the regulation of motivated behavior or the selection of actions based on expected reward. This is achieved thanks to the fact that this area also receives strong inputs from limbic cortical areas and from the amygdala, and it projects to the same areas that the limbic thalamic relay nucleus does (i.e., OFC and PCC). Heroin, for example, is so highly addictive because its binding to receptors of the opioid system produces a massive release of dopamine. Such release in turn causes the individual to feel a strong motivation toward engaging in actions directed toward obtaining the drug. Similarly, though without involving the opioid system, cocaine too "hacks" the dopaminergic system, prompting the user to seek the drug.

The Case of Phineas Gage

Before ending this section on the limbic system, it is worth mentioning the famous case of Phineas Gage, a construction worker who, while working on a railway track in 1848, fell victim to an accidental explosion. The explosion projected a metal bar, which, entering through his eye, pierced his skull and damaged his orbitofrontal cortex. Miraculously, it appeared that nothing serious had happened to the man. At no point did he lose consciousness, memory, perceptual ability, or motility (the damaged area was in the frontal lobe, but far away from the primary motor cortex responsible for activating the muscles). However, the same was not true for Phineas's manners and behavior. Once a responsible and respectful man, following the accident, he became a troublesome and irascible person.

The case of Phineas Gage was one of the first pieces of evidence in history, if not the first, to point to the key role played by the prefrontal cortex, and especially its more ventral parts, in inhibiting impulsive and primitive behaviors when considering their future negative consequences. This is possibly achieved through the close relationship that this area has with the ventral parts of the striatum.

Brain Networks and Neuroimaging Techniques

Integration and Segregation: A Sweet Spot

In order to carry out the functions of perception, evaluation, and action, the fifteen trillion neurons that make up the cerebral cortex must be properly synchronized. Neurons can neither fire all at once, as a single signal could not encode all the richness present in an experience, nor can they fire completely independently of each other, as there would be no integration of information. The first situation occurs during epileptic seizures, while the second occurs when we sleep. Hence, for a conscious experience to occur, certain neurons need to synchronize and form a module that is specialized in processing a specific type of information. Different modules will have different patterns of activity, but, to allow information from one module to reach another and be integrated, connections between them are also necessary. That is, both a certain degree of segregation (obtained through the different modules) and a certain degree of integration (obtained through elements that connect the different modules between them) are required. A schematic representation of this can be found in figure 27.

Functional Magnetic Resonance Imaging (fMRI)

A widely used neuroimaging technique is functional magnetic resonance imaging (fMRI). This technique allows us to measure neuronal activity indirectly by determining oxygen consumption over time in different

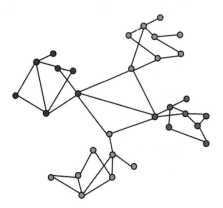

Figure 27. Schematic representation of segregation and integration of information within a system: four different modules (i.e., segregation) are depicted. Connector elements within each module allow the information between them to be integrated.

brain areas. In this technique, the brain is divided into voxels (i.e., three-dimensional pixels), typically three cubic millimeters big. For each voxel in the brain, a time series that captures the levels of activity (Y axis) as time passes (X axis) is obtained. To establish which areas are synchronized, the time series of each voxel is compared with that of all other voxels in the brain, obtaining for each comparison a value that indicates the level of correlation between the signals from both areas. When this value exceeds a threshold set by the researchers, the two areas are considered to work together and belong to the same neural network. By repeating this analysis for each voxel, we can group the different cortical areas into different neural networks. If this analysis is carried out as participants rest inside the scanner without performing any task, we can obtain an approximation to the intrinsic functional architecture of the brain.

Depending on the specific details of the analysis (e.g., the correlation threshold between two areas that the researchers consider indicates that they belong to the same brain network) different groupings can be obtained. After all, the brain is a single interconnected network. However, since this network is not homogeneously connected, we can try to decipher the different functional structures within it.

Yeo Networks

A description of brain networks obtained using functional magnetic resonance imaging widely used in cognitive neuroscience is provided by Randy Buckner's group at Harvard University. Applying complicated analyses, they obtained a description of the brain's functional architecture that establishes that its cortical activity can be grouped into seventeen functional networks, which can, in turn, be regrouped and reduced to seven. Within the scientific community, these are known as the Yeo Networks, named after the lead author of the study, Thomas Yeo.

In figure 28[19] you can see this brain parcellation; to see the figure in color, refer to color plate 11. Be aware that this does not mean that two areas belonging to different networks never coordinate or share information. It just means that they do not do so very often, at least not during

---

19. Image modified from Yeo et al. (2011).

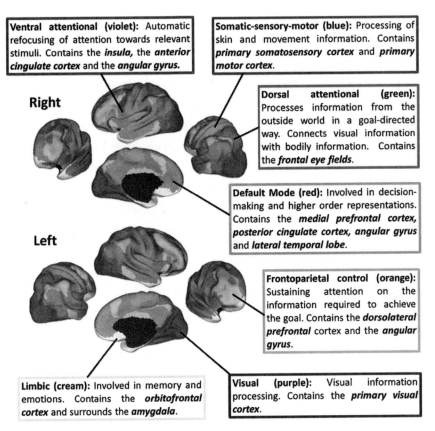

Ventral attentional (violet): Automatic refocusing of attention towards relevant stimuli. Contains the *insula*, the *anterior cingulate cortex* and the *angular gyrus*.

Somatic-sensory-motor (blue): Processing of skin and movement information. Contains *primary somatosensory cortex* and *primary motor cortex*.

Dorsal attentional (green): Processes information from the outside world in a goal-directed way. Connects visual information with bodily information. Contains the *frontal eye fields*.

Default Mode (red): Involved in decision-making and higher order representations. Contains the *medial prefrontal cortex, posterior cingulate cortex, angular gyrus* and *lateral temporal lobe*.

Frontoparietal control (orange): Sustaining attention on the information required to achieve the goal. Contains the *dorsolateral prefrontal* cortex and the *angular gyrus*.

Limbic (cream): Involved in memory and emotions. Contains the *orbitofrontal cortex* and surrounds the *amygdala*.

Visual (purple): Visual information processing. Contains the *primary visual cortex*.

Figure 28. Lateral and medial view of Yeo's functional networks.
(See also color plate 11.)

the resting state. Of course, a very complex interrelationship between the different networks exists that we do not, and neither will we ever, fully understand, especially if we consider the fact that, as we carry out tasks, the connectivity between the areas changes. Nevertheless, these functional groupings are proving to be immensely informative.

The visual network is depicted in purple; the somatic-sensory-motor network, which contains both the primary motor cortex (i.e., the cortical area that directly activates the muscles in charge of executing the action selected by the motor association cortex) and the primary somatosensory cortex (i.e., the area of the cortex that receives the sensory information from the skin and tongue from the somatosensory thalamic relay nucleus) is depicted in blue.

Three neural networks involved in different attentional processes are represented in green, violet, and orange. In an extremely simplified way, we could say that the frontoparietal control network is involved in the maintenance of adequate information in working memory (i.e., short-term memory) during tasks; that the dorsolateral attentional network is responsible for intentionally directing visuospatial attention in a goal-directed manner, connecting the visual cortex with the somatosensory cortex, one of its main areas being the frontal eye fields located in the frontal cortex; and that the ventral attentional network, which is highly involved in the automatic reorientation of attention as a response to the appearance of stimuli relevant to the individual. For this reason, this network is also known as the salience network. Its main hubs are the anterior insula and the anterior cingulate cortex. In yellow you can see the limbic network formed by the orbitofrontal cortex and by the most anterior part of the medial temporal lobe, which surrounds the amygdala. Finally, in red is the default mode network. There is a lot to say about this network.

The Default Mode Network

This network was named the default mode network because it was initially discovered as a set of brain regions whose activity increased precisely when participants were resting as they awaited to begin several laboratory tasks. The areas that form this network consume a lot of energy at all times so their basal activity is very high; however, researchers realized that they would undergo a strong deactivation when starting tasks that required controlled attention. Hence, they called it the task-negative or default mode network. But later, it was pointed out that all the tasks used in the previous discovery required focused attention on the outside world. Instead, when tasks that directed attention to the inner world were employed (e.g., tasks asking the participant to reflect upon whether certain adjectives defined them or not, or tasks that required the activation of autobiographical or social material), it was found that the areas of this network were indeed activated. That is, rather than being a task-negative or resting network, this network seemed to be highly engaged when manipulating internal representations sustained on mnemonic processes, something we do as our minds wander.

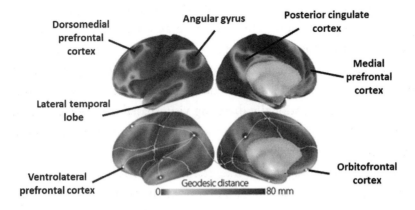

Figure 29. Gradient from the primary cortices to the higher-order integration regions belonging to the default mode network. Image obtained from a study led by Margulies et al. (2016). (See also color plate 12.)

The position of the brain regions that form the default mode network is also quite telling, as it suggests that these regions are located at the end of the integration ladder. This is clearly seen in a collaborative study between the Max Planck Institute and the University of York led by Daniel Margulies and Jonathan Smallwood, with whom I had the pleasure of working during my Ph.D. In this study, complex analyses were carried out that pointed at how the most central regions of the default mode network were located at the maximum cortical equidistance from the primary unimodal zones. This can be seen in color plate 12,[20] which shows a gradient that goes from the unimodal areas of the cortex (sensory and motor), represented in dark blue, to the red areas, which clearly correspond to the areas of the default mode network (see color plate 11).

As indicated by the white lines in the bottom image of color plate 12, the red dots are located at the maximum equidistance from various primary cortices, suggesting that the default

---

20. Image modified from the following article: Margulies DS, Ghosh SS, Goulas A, Falkiewicz M, Huntenburg JM, Langs G, Smallwood J. 2016. Situating the default-mode network along a principal gradient of macroscale cortical organization. Proceedings of the National Academy of Sciences USA 113(44):12574–12579.

mode network represents the maximum point of convergence of information.

This network doesn't only manipulate information from memory. It also contextualizes information from the environment and ultimately decides who we are and how we act. Although as Yeo's parcellation shows, the default mode network can be functionally differentiated from the limbic network, these two networks are highly connected, both anatomically and functionally. Recall that the nuclei of the thalamus involved in limbic functions send projections to the orbitofrontal cortex and the posterior cingulate cortex. Note also that, although Yeo's networks placed the orbitofrontal cortex in the limbic network, in Margulies's analysis, this area appears as one of the areas shown in color plate 12 at the end of the gradient, pointing to the close relationship that the default network has with the limbic system.

The more medial parts of the default mode network, and particularly those located more frontally, are characterized by showing high activation in laboratory tasks that require us to reflect on who we are (for example, by asking us to judge whether or not a series of adjectives presented on the screen define us). In other words, these frontal ends of the default network are highly involved in providing us with an identity. It makes sense that this function is located in the most frontal parts of the motor lobe, for what is our identity if not the construct through which we decide how to behave and interact with the world? It would make sense for this high representation of ourselves to be located in the action-oriented frontal lobe.

Meanwhile, neuroimaging studies using tasks that require semantic manipulation show that the semantic system, which sustains the abstractions acquired through language, is included within the lateral areas of the default mode network, specifically in those located in the temporal lobe and the angular gyrus (figure 29). It is, therefore, logical, that this network is so highly implicated in the mental narrative that occupies our minds as our minds wander. In addition, the angular gyrus, which lies between the visual cortex and the somatosensory cortex, plays an important role in the spatial localization of the self.

Taking all this information into account, we could say that, by sustaining the idea that we have constructed of ourselves, this network is in charge of contextualizing what the representations activated at a given moment, whether internally or externally, mean to us and, based on this meaning, determine the actions that we should execute at any given point in time.

Electroencephalogram (EEG) and Magnetoencephalogram (MEG)

Before concluding this chapter, a brief introduction to electroencephalogram (EEG) and magnetoencephalogram (MEG) is in order, as we will discuss results obtained with these neuroimaging techniques later on in the book.

While functional magnetic resonance imaging (fMRI) measures brain activity indirectly through measuring the oxygen consumption of the different voxels in the brain, EEG and MEG measure brain activity directly by placing sensors around the skull, capable of detecting the electrical currents generated by the brain. Every electrical current has a magnetic field associated with it, and this magnetic field is what MEG detects. EEG, however, detects the electric field. fMRI differs widely from these other techniques in its temporal and spatial resolution. By obtaining information from every voxel within the brain, fMRI has a high spatial resolution (i.e., it tells us very precisely the location where changes in activity or connectivity are occurring). However, this technique has a low temporal resolution, as it only obtains signals every three seconds or so, when processes linked to the nervous system are much faster than this.

In contrast, EEG and MEG can collect signals every 1.5 milliseconds approximately and, therefore, have a high temporal resolution. However, these techniques only collect signals from sensors located on the surface of the brain, so their spatial resolution is highly limited to such sensors. That said, by performing complex analyses, researchers can manage to pinpoint more precisely the origin of the signals detected by the sensors, but even so, its spatial resolution is nowhere as precise as that of functional MRI.

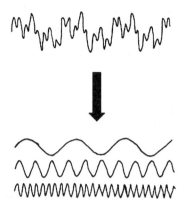

Figure 30. The signal obtained by
a sensor is shown *above*, and the
individual components that make up
that signal, which consist of waves of
different frequencies, are shown *below*.

How are the signals obtained through EEG and MEG analyzed? Many different possibilities exist. A very common analysis consists of breaking down the signals obtained from each sensor into its different components (figure 30), and in doing so, and according to their frequency, obtain waves of a different nature.

In an extremely simplified way, we can say that the slowest frequency waves are the delta waves (associated with deep sleep), followed by the theta waves (associated with rapid eye movement [REM] sleep). These two types of waves seem to originate in the medial temporal lobe. Next are the alpha waves (associated with relaxed wakeful states and top-down information processing), which appear to originate in the midline of the default mode network. Next are beta waves (associated

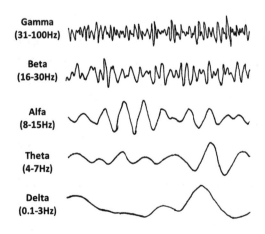

Figure 31. The different
brainwaves according to
their frequency.

with states of alertness), and last are gamma waves (involved in problem solving during cognitive tasks and associated with bottom-up processing) (figure 31).

Summary of Chapter 1
"Understanding Neuroscience"

In this chapter, we have studied the way in which a neuron generates an action potential, how this depends on the balance between positive and negative charges inside the neuron, and how this balance is modulated through the opening or closing of various channels located in the membrane. We have also studied how these channels are regulated by a series of intracellular signals that are often initiated following the binding of a neurotransmitter to membrane receptors, and how a neuron produces only one type of neurotransmitter but has receptors for a multitude of different neurotransmitters, as well as different receptors for the same neurotransmitter.

We have also talked about neuroplasticity. Namely, about how, through incorporating or eliminating receptors from the postsynaptic neuron's synaptic boutons, synaptic strengths are modulated according to the frequency by which a synapse occurs. We have studied how learning or forgetting depends on this mechanism, which ultimately endows with great fluidity the synaptic strength map that forms our model, thereby allowing life experience to constantly update it.

We have also studied the anatomical organization of the cerebral cortex and how sensory information travels from the sensory organs to the cortex, becoming more and more integrated as it passes from unimodal to association areas, finally reaching the default mode network, thanks to both horizontal (i.e., cortico-cortical) and vertical (i.e., between the cortex and subcortical structures) projections.

We have learned how, as bottom-up information ascends to become more and more integrated, it is compared with top-down information contained in the higher-order models we have created of the world. When a discordance between the bottom-up and the top-down information is detected, a prediction error is generated that allows only new information to ascend and be incorporated to update the model. In a continuous cycle, this new updated model will now, in turn, be used to compare with new ascending bottom-up information (the theory of hierarchical predictive coding).

We have emphasized that the brain is an organ involved in a constant cycle of perception-evaluation-action and that the evaluation of information takes place in the limbic system, which is responsible for comparing incoming information with information from memory and deciding whether the current stimulus represents a reward or a threat. And according to this cycle, the prefrontal cortex will select the appropriate action to take.

Finally, we have learned that brain activity is organized into functional networks formed by highly synchronized areas that give rise to distinct and relatively stable spatiotemporal patterns. We also learned that the default mode network not only contains the brain areas that consume the most energy, but being located at the end of the integration ladder, is also involved in functions unique to human beings, such as language and identity.

In short, we have studied the sensory world, the emotional world, and the world of ideas, three worlds that, as we will see further on, are highly affected during the psychedelic experience.

References for Further Study

Beliveau V, Ganz M, Feng L, Ozenne B, Højgaard L, Fisher PM, Svarer C, Greve DN, Knudsen, GM. 2017. A high-resolution in vivo atlas of the human brain's serotonin system. Journal of Neuroscience 37(1):120–128.

Buckner RL, Krienen FM. 2013. The evolution of distributed association networks in the human brain. Trends in Cognitive Sciences 17(12):648–665.

Edelman GM, Tononi G. 2008. A universe of consciousness: how matter becomes imagination. London: Hachette UK.

Margulies DS, Ghosh SS, Goulas A, Falkiewicz M, Huntenburg JM, Langs G, Bezgin G, Eickhoff SB, Castellanos FX, Petrides M, et al. 2016. Situating the default-mode network along a principal gradient of macroscale cortical organization. Proceedings of the National Academy of Sciences USA 113(44):12574–12579.

Nadal MS, Amarillo Y. El tálamo en el centro de la atención [The thalamus in the center of attention]. 2018. Ciencia Hoy [Science Today] 27(160):36–40.

Shipp S. 2016. Neural elements for predictive coding. Frontiers in Psychology 7:1792.

Yeo BT, Krienen FM, Sepulcre J, Sabuncu MR, Lashkari D, Hollinshead M, Roffman JL, Smoller JW, Zöllei L, Polimeni JR, et al. 2011. The organization of the human cerebral cortex estimated by intrinsic functional connectivity. Journal of Neurophysiology 106(5):2322–45.

2

Using Psychoactives
in Therapy

Before delving into the possible mechanisms underlying the therapeutic effects that classic psychedelics and MDMA appear to have, we must review the current state of the clinical research.

The truth is that the current scientific evidence still stands at a rather preliminary stage, considering medicine's usual standards. Even in the most recent and biggest studies, the sample sizes are small and this is not the only criticism that a skeptic could make.

As we shall see, all clinical studies have found a significant improvement in symptoms. It is however important to note that, except for the first ayahuasca study, the punctual use of the psychoactive drug was embedded within a prolonged therapeutic process that both preceded the psychoactive session and continued after it. In research, control groups are exposed to the same conditions as the experimental group, with exception of the intervention being researched, in this case, the induced altered state of consciousness. In the case of psychedelics, most studies haven't included a control group. Without this group, it is therefore impossible to discern which aspects of the symptoms' improvement were due to the altered state of consciousness itself from those due to the therapeutic context or to the participants' expectations.

Having said this, the most recent studies do contain a control group; and even though, as of today, few data are still available, the results obtained so far suggest that including such altered states of consciousness within the therapeutic process, may significantly accelerate symptom improvement.

Furthermore, although many studies did not include a control group, many of them found that the reported intensity of the experience predicted the magnitude of the obtained benefits. This also suggests that there's something unique about the psychedelic experience that contributes to the healing process.

A skeptic could also criticize that participants were carefully selected through detailed interviews. During these interviews, the therapists, guided by their "clinical eye," could use subjective criteria, or participants with whom they felt they could quickly build a strong therapeutic alliance, given the short period of time available to work together during clinical trials. Strict exclusion and inclusion criteria were also employed during the selection process. For example, all studies excluded people with a psychotic or bipolar disorder, and clinical trials using classic psychedelics also excluded those with suicidal ideation. Thus, the participants in the studies were in no way selected randomly. We should therefore apply extreme caution when extrapolating these results to the entire population. It would be unwise to assume that, had participants been selected less selectively, results would have been equally positive. Future research will have to explore this in more detail. What percentage of people can truly benefit from such altered states of consciousness?

The few results available from the samples studied, however, are so promising that many people, psychiatrists included, have dared to affirm that the use of these molecules within psychotherapeutic contexts will revolutionize psychiatry. In light of the results obtained so far, it is undeniable that governments, psychiatrists, and psychotherapists around the globe should cease to ignore the possible therapeutic potential of these substances. Governments should reclassify them as soon as possible and start facilitating the advancement of research. Thankfully, we can already see some glimpses of this research. For example, several governments, such as those from Australia and the United States, have already begun funding research into these therapies, and in 2024 the European Union announced funding 6.5 million euros for the PsyPal clinical trial focused on studying the use of psilocybin to treat psychological distress in people facing an incurable illness requiring palliative care. Moreover, to accelerate research, both psychedelic-assisted therapy for treatment-resistant and major depression, and MDMA-assisted therapy for post-traumatic stress disorder, have been granted "breakthrough therapy" status by the North American Food and Drug Administration (FDA). As we shall soon see, this is because many of the participants included in the clinical studies that positively responded to this treatment had previously failed to respond to other psychiatric and psychotherapeutic interventions. Most likely we will see major advances within this field in the coming years.

That being said, classic psychedelics such as LSD and psilocybin are not necessarily helpful for every psychopathology. In fact, in some cases, they can be dangerous and extremely destabilizing. However, at present, it does seem as if the altered states of consciousness that they promote could have certain therapeutic potential to improve symptoms in unipolar major depression (in contrast to bipolar depression in which there's a fluctuation between depression and euphoria), reduce anxiety linked to life-threatening diseases, combat addictive behaviors, and improve symptoms present in obsessive-compulsive disorder. But we must be cautious. Successfully navigating an experience of this sort requires a certain attitude and preparation, even within controlled settings. Despite the fact that psychedelic-assisted therapy might be able to help many people suffering from these disorders, it won't necessarily always be the solution, neither at any moment in time nor for everyone.

Regarding MDMA-assisted therapy, as we shall see, studies have mainly focused on patients suffering from a post-traumatic stress disorder, and once again, results suggest that this type of intervention has powerful therapeutic potential. Preliminary studies have also been conducted for other psychopathologies beyond post-traumatic stress disorder, namely, social anxiety in autistic individuals and alcohol addiction.

Both types of psychoactive-assisted therapies (i.e., using classic psychedelics and using MDMA) being applied in clinical trials share some aspects and differ in others. In both cases, preparation sessions precede the psychoactive session. During these preparatory sessions, the participants are informed about the effects they might feel during the altered state and the way in which the psychoactive session will be conducted. They are also given tips regarding how to best navigate the experience. Namely, they are informed about the importance of surrendering to the experience, letting go, and trusting in the molecule's ability to guide the process. Importantly, these sessions also offer the therapists an opportunity to build a therapeutic alliance and get to know the participants' problems and fears. This is key, as it will allow the participant to feel safe and supported as they explore and face their emotions during the altered state of consciousness.

In both types of therapies, psychoactive sessions are also followed by several integration sessions. These sessions are aimed at discussing, providing meaning to, and integrating into consciousness as well as into everyday life, the content that popped up during the altered state of consciousness. To achieve this outcome, other techniques beyond talking can be used, namely, techniques that promote artistic expression, such as drawing, dancing, and writing. Therapists insist on how, to achieve long-lasting benefits, an active effort of integrating the experience must be made by the individual the days following the experience. Throughout the therapeutic process, the participant is usually accompanied by a team of two therapists. Generally, one is female and the other one male, providing safety both to the participants and to the therapists. The specific therapeutic style employed outside of the psychoactive session varies throughout the studies since the style has to adapt to both the psychopathology being treated and to the therapists' expertise. For example, addiction studies have employed motivational therapy or cognitive behavioral therapy; some depression studies have employed acceptance and commitment therapy, and the MDMA study with autistic individuals has employed mindfulness-based therapy adapted from dialectical behavior therapy.

The Multidisciplinary Association for Psychedelic Studies (MAPS) has developed a manual, which, despite being focused primarily on MDMA-assisted psychotherapy, also applies in a fundamental way to psychedelic-assisted psychotherapy. On top of providing the reader with the necessary information regarding both the preparation and integration sessions, this manual specifies the way in which the psychoactive sessions should be conducted. Given its high potential to evoke emotions, participants are always accompanied by music during these sessions. Such music should adjust well to what the participant is experiencing on a moment-to-moment basis. Hence, the therapists must have prepared a musical playlist in advance and be well familiar with it.

Given the phenomenological differences between classic psychedelics and MDMA (we will study them throughout the book), during psychoactive sessions with classic psychedelics, participants are invited to go inward and explore their feelings and perceptions throughout the entire session, whereas during MDMA sessions, moments of internal exploration are combined with moments of discussion with the therapists. Despite this difference, rigid formulas must always be avoided and therapists must, instead, try to adapt to the needs of the specific moment and the specific participant.

The therapeutic protocols applied with both molecules thus far differ in some additional aspects besides the internal versus external focus during the psychoactive session. In general, MDMA-assisted therapies last longer than psychedelic-assisted ones. However, protocols have varied even within the same molecule. During the MDMA studies, participants generally consume three to four high doses of MDMA (one per month) and receive three to four integration sessions in between. In clinical studies using classic psychedelics, participants commonly receive two increasingly higher doses separated, approximately, by only a week or two. In some studies the doses applied in both sessions were moderately perceptible, whereas in others only the second session used perceptible doses. Three doses or, in contrast, a single perceptible dose have also been used on some occasions. The ultimate protocol is still being devised and it is likely to vary depending on the participants' characteristics.

Despite the differences between both substances, a central component of MAPS' therapeutic approach is the belief that, just as a physical wound tends to heal itself when disinfected, the psyche also tends to heal when it feels cared for. It is therefore essential that both participants and therapists trust that a healing intelligence lies within us. A healing force that is aided by the psychoactive drug will guide the participants toward that which they need to experience in order to heal. Therefore, both during the preparation and the psychoactive sessions themselves, the participant is told, and reminded, of the importance of trusting that the emergence of difficult emotions is an integral part of the healing process. Hence, instead of rejecting them and trying to suppress those difficult emotions, they should try to, with openness and curiosity, invite them into the experience and explore what it is that the difficult emotions might be offering. They must also be reminded that the sole role of the therapists is to accompany and support them throughout the process and that they will be safe and secure at all times.

Following the theory of inner healing intelligence, psychoactive sessions should not be directed by the therapists. Instead, they should try to allow for the participant to find the answers by themselves, the main role of the therapist being to offer company and security and, at all times, demonstrate an empathic presence. Nonetheless, if after a prolonged period of time, therapists perceive that the participant, for example, is deviating from processing the trauma (something extremely rare) or they feel like the participant could benefit from a certain comment, they can intervene, if needed, by suggesting something to redirect the participant. The participant could, for example, start paying excessive attention to the distorted visual inputs coming in from the external world. As fascinating and beautiful as the external world can seem, this externally-oriented attention could be distracting the participant from going inwards, so after some time of such external exploration, the therapist could suggest shifting the exploration inwards. The therapists must always allow the altered state of consciousness to provide the participant with the information he or she needs but, ultimately, an optimal middle ground between acting as an empathic and passive companion and facilitating the session must be met. Hence, the therapists must apply the intuition acquired throughout their professional experience, as well as their expertise regarding the substance they are working with.

Therapists conducting therapies that involve altered states of consciousness must also be familiar with the possibility of traumas expressing themselves through the body. Hence, they should know how to apply somatic therapies that work with energetic blockages, such as body scans of breathing techniques. They should also be aware that participants might have a transpersonal experience of a spiritual, psychic, or perinatal nature during a session. Such experiences might challenge the materialistic and rational worldview of the West and should never be pathologized nor judged negatively.

Finally, the perception of one's psyche being comprised of many different parts is frequently experienced during these altered states of consciousness. The realization that our whole being goes far beyond our damaged parts and that these damaged parts of us are just trying to play a specific role, often aimed at protecting us, can be extremely helpful, since it can help us accept and integrate them into their consciousness. Therapists working with altered states of consciousness should therefore be familiar with this understanding of the psyche. Hence, therapies such as internal family systems or voice dialogue, which understand the psyche through this multiplicity, will be highly compatible with altered states of consciousness-assisted therapy.

After briefly reviewing how these therapies are conducted, it's time to review in detail the results obtained when applying them. This way, without forgetting about the aforementioned limitations, you will be able to draw your own conclusions regarding their therapeutic potential. You will probably realize that these are not miracle molecules, but that, in certain situations, they do seem to be useful tools.

Psychedelic-Assisted Therapy

In the following section, we will study the different clinical applications being studied in clinical trials using, on one hand, a series of classic psychedelics, and on the other hand, using MDMA. We will see how clinical trials on depression have mainly focused on using psilocybin, whereas treatment of post-traumatic stress disorder has mainly focused on MDMA. However, we will also see how the same condition has been treated with different classical psychedelics, such as substance use disorders and emotional distress linked to a terminal diagnosis, which have been treated with both psilocybin and LSD. And similarly, in addition to classic psychedelics, MDMA has also shown potential for treating alcohol addiction. Ultimately, it is likely that these substances work in a rather transdiagnostic way, whereby the same substance can be used to treat a variety of conditions, and the same condition can be treated by diverse substances. In this chapter we will focus on the main clinical applications that have been studied so far for each substance, but as clinical trials start exploring more substances and more psychopathologies, the current substance-psychopathology pairing presented below is likely to change.

Depression—Ayahuasca and Psilocybin

A group from the University of São Paulo led by Jorge Hallak conducted one of the first preliminary studies of psychedelics and depression in 2016 using an ayahuasca preparation cooked by members of the Santo Daime community.

Ayahuasca is an Amazonian brew used by shamans from Indigenous communities to enter the spirit world in order to communicate and battle different energies within that realm, often done with healing purposes. Multiple variations of this cocktail exist, which hinders our ability to carry out rigorous clinical research that can be easily replicated; however, given the current explosion of people traveling to the Amazon in search of this experience, it is worth mentioning something about this Amazonian brew.

Despite its many variations, ayahuasca's main ingredient is a plant called *Banisteriopsis caapi*. This plant is non-psychedelic and is often mixed with another psychoactive plant called *Psychotria viridis*, which contains the potent psychedelic dimethyltryptamine (DMT).

Despite *B. caapi* being non-psychedelic, Indigenous people still seem to believe that it holds medicinal power. When modern science has studied the contents within this plant, it has found that it contains a series of alkaloids that have the peculiar ability to act as enzyme inhibitors. Namely, these alkaloids belong to the family of harmala alkaloids which inhibit MAO[1] enzymes, highly involved in digestion and metabolic processes.

---

1. Monoamine oxidases (MAO).

Following on from the medicinal claims made by the Amazonian people, curious researchers in the West have conducted several pre-clinical studies to explore the potential antidepressant and neurogenic effects of these non-psychedelic MAO inhibiting alkaloids, finding rather extraordinary results that suggest that these alkaloids might be holding some of the secrets behind the medicinal properties claimed by the Indigenous people.

First, in 2006 a study by Farzin and Mansouri from Mazandaran University of Medical Sciences in Iran found that these alkaloids elicited antidepressant-like effects during a mouse swim test, where depression levels were calculated based on the time the mouse spent trying to escape the water tank before giving up. The antidepressant effects of these alkaloids were then replicated using both chronic and acute administration by two studies from 2010 and 2009, respectively, led by Jucélia Fortunato, from Universidade do Extremo Sul Catarinense, Brazil. Not only were behavioral antidepressant effects found with both chronic and acute administrations, but Fortunato's studies also found increased levels of a protein involved in neuronal growth (brain-derived neurotrophic factor [BDNF]), in the hippocampus, a key region involved in the encoding and retrieval of information that is highly connected to the default mode network through the limbic relay nuclei of the thalamus. The hippocampus also contains one of the only regions of the brain capable of birthing new neurons: the subgranular zone. In these regions, progenitor cells can proliferate, differentiate, and mature into different neural cells such as neurons, astrocytes,[2] or microglia.[3]

To study whether *B. caapi*'s alkaloids could induce neurogenesis in these regions, Jordi Riba's group, from Sant Pau Institute of Biomedical Research, in a study led by Jose A. Morales-García from Complutense

---

2. Astrocytes are the most prevalent cell type in the nervous system. They are non-neural cells (i.e., they don't fire action potentials) and they provide neurons with diverse forms of support. For example, they provide them with glucose and mitocondria, and they maintain the extracellular ion balance.

3. Microglia are the immune cells in the nervous system in charge of the defense mechanisms.

University de Madrid, took progenitor cells[4] from the subgranular zone of an adult rat's hippocampus and prepared cell cultures with them. More specifically, they prepared neurospheres, which are a special type of cell culture, where free-floating clusters of stem cells (in this case the progenitor cells from the subgranular zone) are suspended in a medium that contains the necessary growth factors to survive and proliferate. In these neurosphere cell cultures, cells are suspended because the substrate in which they grow lacks adherent molecules. This allows the progenitor cells to grow into three-dimensional shapes, different from the original two-dimensional cell cultures where cells grow on a flat surface.

The progenitor cells in this study were treated with the different alkaloids and after several days, those cultures treated with the *B. caapi* alkaloids not only presented a higher number of neurospheres, suggesting protective properties that allowed more progenitor cells to survive, but the diameter of these neurospheres was also significantly bigger than those neurospheres in the basal condition where no alkaloids were received. These alkaloids certainly seem to be promoting cell proliferation!

In addition to measuring the neurosphere's size and number, Riba's team also studied cell proliferation and cell differentiation within the neurospheres using fluorescent agents that only bind to molecules found in certain cells types, demonstrating that the administration of the *B. caapi* alkaloids significantly increased not only the proliferation of new stem cells, but also their differentiation into both neurons and astrocytes, thus acting as potent neurogenic agents. This effect was not only found in cell cultures developed from progenitor cells taken from the subgranular zone of the hippocampus. It was also found in progenitor cells taken from another region capable of producing neurogenesis (the subventricular zone). Morales-García recently shared with me how he repeated the experiments several times before publishing them because he couldn't believe the magnitude of the effect! It certainly looks as if

---

4. Progenitor cells are multipotent cells that can proliferate, meaning that they can divide and produce new cells that have the ability to mature into several different cells types according to the signals received from the environment.

the Indigenous communities are onto something when assigning medicinal properties to these non-psychedelic MAO inhibiting plants!

But there's more! In addition to the incredible neurogenic properties found in *B. caapi*, it turns out that without this plant, the DMT from *P. viridis* would be degraded by the MAO enzymes located in our gastrointestinal tract before reaching our brain! How Indigenous communities came up with the synergic combination of these two plants is a mystery to the Western mind! Some may say it was through trial and error; however, legends have it that it was the plants themselves who communicated this information to the Indigenous people.

Unlike Western psychiatrists and psychologists, shamanic cultures have been accumulating knowledge pertaining to the appropriate use of their plant medicines for centuries. While the peculiarities of our Western cosmovision should be taken into account as we in the West try to integrate these medicines into our society, there surely is a lot that we can learn from Indigenous peoples. The epistemological approach that Indigenous people use might be different to that of Western society, but ultimately, both approaches seem to produce valuable knowledge systems. In this respect, Onaya Science is an independent research organization working along with the Shipibo-Konibo people in a quest to study the parallels and differences between the two knowledge systems and, where possible, to translate Indigenous knowledge into Western biomedical terms.

Although the shamanic use of psychedelics is beyond the scope of this book, we will briefly mention how, like in the Western model, in shamanic cultures the idea of preparation and integration also exists but mostly consists of following certain diets, avoiding busy environments, and abstaining from drugs and sex for a few weeks before and after the ceremony, rather than the one-to-one psychotherapy sessions employed in Western clinical trials.[5] However, despite their differences, both models have a therapeutic intention behind them. This said, "ayahuasca tourism" has spawned a multitude of false shamans, whose intentions, far from revolving around healing, instead revolve around money and

---

5. Group integration sessions are also being conducted in the West, but are not part of the protocols developed in current clinical trials.

power. If you wish to have an experience in this kind of retreat setting, it is recommended that you choose your shaman carefully, since during the psychedelic experience you will find yourself in an extremely vulnerable position. Not feeling safe and well accompanied could have fatal consequences and there have been quite a few reported cases of sexual abuse. Be careful who you trust![6] Unfortunately, cases of sexual misconduct have also been reported in some of the clinical trials, where therapists take advantage of their clients' vulnerable state. This is something to really watch out for as the Psychedelic Renaissance develops.

In terms of ayahuasca in the context of clinical trials, the preliminary 2016 ayahuasca study by Halak's team mentioned above included seventeen people suffering from recurrent depression. Most of them were moderately depressed, and all had recently withdrawn from previous treatments due to a lack of positive results. When the group's depressive symptoms were measured three weeks after the psychedelic session, they had more than halved. An initial baseline mean score of 19.24, corresponding to moderate levels of depression (according to the Hamilton scale, commonly used to measure depressive symptoms), turned into a mean score of 7.56, corresponding to mild depression. The results were statistically significant.

Occurring in parallel, another study was being carried out at Imperial College London by David Nutt's group. In this 2018 study, led by Robin Carhart-Harris, psilocybin, an active component present in the "magic" mushrooms of the genus *Psilocybe*, was used instead of ayahuasca. Because psilocybin concentrations vary from one mushroom to another, and because medical research standards require absolute control of the applied doses administered, the psilocybin molecules used in research are now being synthesized in the laboratory[7] (i.e., participants do not ingest the mushrooms). Reducing the intake to a single molecule and controlling the dose to the milligram certainly improves scientific

6. Some websites can help you find a good trip sitter or a good retreat center. For example, Tripsitters, Psilocybin Community & Education Hub; Psychedelic Therapy, Primal Nature; or AyaAdvisors, Ayahuasca Retreat Reviews.

7. For this study, psilocybin was synthesized at the pharmaceutical laboratory of Guy's and St. Thomas' Hospital in London.

rigor, but it is worth mentioning that it, too, increases in a significant way the research expenses.

In addition to the psychoactive substances employed, another significant difference between the two first studies on depression is that in the ayahuasca study conducted by Hallak, participants received no preparatory or integrative therapy sessions with the person(s) who was to be their chaperones during the hallucinogenic experience. Instead, in the study carried out by the Imperial College London (and in all subsequent clinical trials published up to 2024), there was psychological support before, during, and after the psychedelic treatment. More specifically, in Carhart-Harris's study, patients had a four-hour-long intensive preparatory session with those therapists that would accompany them during the psilocybin intake. Additionally, the psychoactive treatment consisted of two escalating doses of psilocybin separated by a week. The first one consisted of 10 mg (a low but perceptible dose), and the second one consisted of 25 mg, considered a moderate dose. As for the integration sessions, only a telephone call to monitor any adverse effects was made the day after the low dose. After the higher dose, the participants had two face-to-face sessions aimed at integrating the psychedelic experience: one the following day, and one a week later.

If you search Spotify for "Psilodep Session 2" you can find one of the playlists used by Nutt's team in the psychedelic sessions with depressed patients. Although musical tastes are extremely subjective, certain guidelines can be followed when creating a playlist for this purpose. For example, the intensity of the music should follow a similar dynamic to the intensity of the psychedelic experience, which, in the case of psilocybin, peaks two to three hours after intake.

The inclusion criteria for this study involved having failed at least two different pharmacological treatments (during the same depressive episode) and to be suffering from severe or moderate unipolar depression. Twenty participants took part in the study. Eighteen of them found relief from severe depression and the remaining two found relief from moderate depression.

What did Nutt's team find? Firstly, it found that psilocybin use under these therapeutic conditions was generally well tolerated by participants. Acceptable levels of anxiety, confusion, nausea, and headache (and, in two cases, moments of mild paranoia during the peak of the experience), were found in only a few cases.

Depressive symptoms were measured before the psychedelic treatment and six times afterward, the last measurement being taken six months after the psychedelic experience (figure 32). By the first week, results showed that all participants had responded significantly to the psychedelic experience. However, in general, symptoms seemed to eventually return. At week five, four participants were in remission, but a significant response was maintained only in nine of them. When depressive symptoms were measured again after six months, only three of these nine participants had relapsed. Ultimately, the results showed that, although the abrupt improvement in symptoms observed immediately after treatment lost momentum over time, at the six-month time point, the group still showed an overall statistically significant reduction in depressive symptoms.

There was no control group for this study, so it was impossible to discern those therapeutic effects specifically caused by psilocybin from those due to the psychological support received during the study. Nevertheless, the results are particularly striking when one considers that this group of participants had been depressed for an average of seventeen years. Additionally, a mean of four previous treatments had failed them in the past. Anxious symptoms were also measured at the six-month time point, and a significant reduction in these was also

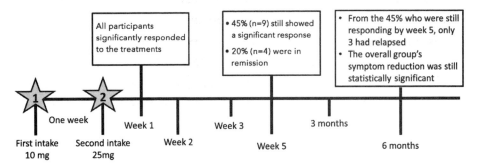

Figure 32. Timing of data collection and results of the 2018 study led by Robin Carhart-Harris.

found. Despite its major limitations due to its being only a preliminary study, the results were definitely encouraging.

Another study published in 2021 on patients with moderate to severe major depression carried out by Ronald Griffiths's team from Johns Hopkins University found similar results.

As in the previous study by Imperial College, in the Johns Hopkins study, led by Alan K. Davis, participants received preparation sessions during the three weeks prior to the psychedelic session; two psychedelic sessions with increasing doses, separated by an average of one and a half weeks; and integration sessions after the psychedelic experience (figure 33). However, in this study, both doses were moderately high (instead of using consecutive doses of 10 mg and 25 mg, they used 20 mg and 30 mg). When comparing depressive symptoms right before the preparatory session to those four weeks after the second psychedelic session, researchers not only found that the symptoms had halved in 71 percent of the patients, but 54 percent of them were in remission! In this case, the sample consisted of twenty-four participants who, on average, had been suffering from depression for 21.5 years, having been trapped in the current major depressive episode for one year. Once again, the sample size was very small, participants had been carefully selected, and there was no control group, but given the characteristics of the group, it is not unreasonable to think that some people can indeed benefit from psychedelic-assisted therapy.

The recurring problem regarding the absence of a control group was finally tackled in a 2023 study conducted by Compass Pathways, a company focused on the development of psychedelic therapies. The sample size was also improved in this study. This study, which was led by Guy Goodwin, consisted of a total of two hundred thirty-three patients with treatment-resistant depression, which were divided into three different groups. One group of seventy-five participants received a 10-mg dose of psilocybin, while another group of seventy-nine participants received a 25-mg dose. Finally, a third group, also consisting of seventy-nine patients, acted as a control group, receiving a placebo dose of 1 mg of psilocybin.

As in the previous psilocybin studies, all participants received psychological support. In particular, the participants had three preparatory

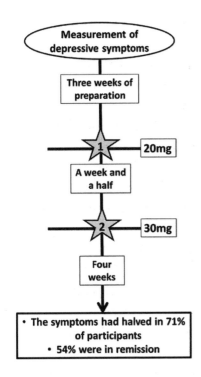

Figure 33. Timing and results of the Johns Hopkins University group's study. Stars indicate days of psilocybin intake.

sessions with their assigned therapists before the psychedelic session, and three integration sessions afterward. The first integration session took place the day after the psychedelic session and the second integration session a week later, each lasting an hour and a half. Finally, after twelve weeks, they had one last, thirty-minute-long session.

Depressive symptoms were measured the day before and the day after taking psilocybin, and weekly during the next twelve weeks. A significant response to treatment was considered only when symptoms were reduced by at least half. The results showed that by the twelfth week, twice as many participants on the 25-mg dose group had had a significant response compared to the control group. At the third week time point, 29 percent of the 25-mg group were in remission[8] compared to only 7.6 percent of the control group, almost four times as many people! And after twelve weeks, 26.6 percent of that group were still in remission, compared to only 11.4 percent of the control group.

8. Being in remission means that scores on depression scales are no longer considered indicative of depression.

There were, however, no statistically significant differences between the participants taking the 10-mg dose and the control group. This study, therefore, provided valuable information regarding the dosage required to obtain benefits. The results also suggest that a single high dose of psilocybin is sufficient to achieve significant therapeutic improvements.

Importantly, the fact that during this study all three groups received the same psychological support seems to be a strong indicator that the reduction of depressive symptoms is significantly due to the psychedelic experience.

Despite these promising results, we should not ignore that such results also reflect the fact that psychedelic-assisted therapy does not significantly help all participants, and that, when it does, its effects are not always sustained indefinitely. Now that psychedelic-assisted therapy is reaching the mainstream, it is essential to emphasize that every patient is different. We must be especially careful as to not create expectations that do not match reality. Such a mistake could lead to a profound disappointment in those people who do not benefit from this therapy, a disappointment which may, in turn, lead to an increase in suicidal ideation and behavior in people who are already in an extremely vulnerable and unstable situation. Psychotherapists should learn to differentiate between the patients likely to benefit from such therapy and those who are not, and to always warn against having too high expectations.

This being said, in a conversation on James W. Jesso's podcast *Adventures through the Mind*, Rosalind Watts, clinical leader of the Imperial College's clinical trials on depression, recounts how, according to some patients' statements, although depression does tend to recur in the long run (note that the studies involve patients who have spent a substantial part of their lives depressed), the psychedelic experience does seem to teach them new ways of relating and reacting to their symptoms.

Comparing Psilocybin to Conventional Antidepressants

How does the effectiveness of the psychedelic experience compare with that of other antidepressants? Based on previous studies, in which this type of therapy helped people for whom other drug treatments had failed, one might suspect that the psychedelic experience is more effective than other conventional alternatives. Is this necessarily always the case?

To address this question, Imperial College London conducted a study in which, for the first and, so far, only time, the reduction in depressive symptoms between a group receiving high-dose psilocybin-assisted therapy was directly compared to that of another group receiving escitalopram-assisted therapy. Escitalopram is one of the most widely used and effective conventional antidepressants, which, unlike psychedelics, produce slow and subtle changes in the psyche. This antidepressant is a selective serotonin reuptake inhibitor (SSRI). That is, it exerts its action by inhibiting the serotonin reuptake protein located in the membrane of the axon terminal of presynaptic neurons. Remember that these proteins are responsible for reintroducing the neurotransmitter released by the presynaptic neuron back into the neuron, thus clearing up the synaptic space. By inhibiting these proteins, this drug lengthens the duration of serotonin in the synaptic space, thereby lengthening its effect on the postsynaptic neuron. This, in turn, promotes long-term changes in the expression of receptors located on the membrane, ultimately affecting the patient's mental state.

In this study, each group consisted of thirty participants. Those in the escitalopram group took this antidepressant daily for six weeks, whereas the psilocybin group took a daily placebo pill for the six weeks. Additionally, the latter group took a high dose of psilocybin at the beginning of the intervention followed by another one, three weeks later. On those same days, patients in the escitalopram group received a minimal and unnoticeable dose of psilocybin (1 mg). The sole purpose of this was to match the two conditions as closely as possible so that the psychedelic experience would be the only difference between both groups. After ingesting the psilocybin, patients were accompanied by their respective psychotherapists for about six hours while music played in the background.

In addition to the pharmacological treatment, patients had important psychological support during the study. Its therapeutic contribution cannot be ignored. There were two preparation sessions. The first one lasted one hour and was conducted on the same day that the patients were informed about being accepted in the study. The second one took place the day before the first psilocybin dose and lasted three hours. The integration sessions took place during the weeks corresponding to, and immediately after, the psilocybin intake. Additionally, during the six weeks that the study lasted, participants met with psychotherapists weekly for conventional therapy (i.e., therapist-directed therapy, no music, no psilocybin).

What did the study find? Is psilocybin truly a better adjunct to psychological support than escitalopram?

The relatively encouraging results from previous studies, in which psychedelic-assisted therapy had succeeded where other treatments had failed, had set high expectations. However, the results obtained in this latest study did not live up to them. Depressive symptoms were measured just before the first psychedelic session, and seven more times over the following six weeks, with both groups showing a marked decrease in symptoms after the first psilocybin-music session. This decline was sustained over the six weeks of the study, and while there was a trend toward greater symptom improvement in the psilocybin group, the difference between both groups was not statistically significant.

While not living up to the immense expectations that had been set for this therapy, the results are nonetheless encouraging. After all, it seems that psilocybin is at least as effective as a well-established antidepressant, at least during the first six weeks of treatment. Moreover, unlike SSRIs, which require daily dosing, psilocybin required only occasional dosing, a definite bonus for this novel treatment. Importantly, psilocybin does not produce the debilitating side effects commonly associated with SSRIs, such as ongoing nausea and dizziness. In this particular study, patients treated with escitalopram were found to have higher levels of anxiety, sexual dysfunction, dry mouth, and lower emotional responsiveness than those treated with psilocybin.

Psilocybin in Combination with SSRIs

Up until 2023, all psychedelic studies on depression had been conducted on patients who, either because they had just completed an ineffective treatment or because they had been required to stop their treatment in order to participate in the psilocybin trials, were not taking antidepressants. The reason for this was that, up until then, a negative interaction between psychedelics and antidepressants had been suspected. Depending on the specific antidepressant, this interaction could, at best, inhibit the action of the psychedelic, and, at worst, be life threatening. For this reason, the studies mentioned so far exploring the treatment of psychedelics for depression had excluded anyone taking antidepressants.

Although conventional antidepressants are unable to address the root of the problem and often fail to cure depression, they can reduce the patient's emotional distress, making depression more manageable. Hence, even if conventional antidepressants do not cure depression, abandoning their treatments in order to try this new therapy is a huge challenge for many patients. In the case of serotonin reuptake inhibitors such as escitalopram, it was suspected that the potential interaction could only diminish the effects of psychedelics, but not cause a health hazard to the individual. To find out whether, to benefit from psychedelic-assisted therapy, abandoning this pharmacological treatment was truly necessary, the next crucial step was to investigate whether or not psilocybin treatment was compatible with this type of antidepressant.

Two studies exploring potential interactions between classic psychedelics and SSRIs have been published. The first study was conducted by a Swiss group led by Matthias Liechti and explored potential interactions between psilocybin and the SSRI Escitalopram in twenty three healthy people, finding few subjective differences during the psychedelic experience between participants who, for seven days before the full psilocybin dose, had received a pretreatment of Escitalopram versus those who had received a placebo. These results on healthy people were the first to suggest that no major interactions exist between these molecules. Following this 2021 study on healthy people, in 2023 Compass Pathways published another study where, for the first time, participants suffering from depression were not tapered off from their SSRI treatments before receiving the psychedelic-assisted therapy. This study, which was led by Guy Goodwin, found similar results to those published in 2023 by this same company on patients who had withdrawn from their SSRI treatment prior to receiving psilocybin. Results so far seem to suggest that treatment with SSRI-type antidepressants does not interfere with the antidepressant effects of psilocybin. The treatment also seems to reduce some of the negative effects commonly associated with the psychedelic experience, such as feelings of anxiety that can occur. Importantly, in September 2023 Small Pharma, another biotech company from London exploring the question of psychedelic-antidepressant interactions, reported some very interesting results that have not yet been published. In this case they were testing intravenous DMT instead of psilocybin and found that participants on SSRIs had even better responses to the DMT treatment than those without them!

This set of discoveries will likely mark a turning point in psychedelic research on the treatment of depression. First of all, it will ease the recruitment process by increasing the number of participants available for the studies. Secondly, people suffering from depression who have been on SSRI medication for some time may soon be able to access psilocybin-assisted therapy without having to face the anguish of coming off antidepressants first.

Cancer or Terminal Illness Diagnosis—LSD and Psilocybin

If psychedelic-assisted therapy can reduce depressive symptoms in people who have experienced them for years, is it possible that psychedelic-assisted therapy could also improve the quality of life of people who, due to a diagnosis of terminal illness, suffer from high levels of anxiety and depression?

Several studies were carried out as early as the 1950s and 1960s that pointed in this direction. At that time, the studies were carried out using LSD, the molecule that Albert Hofmann had serendipitously discovered. At Spring Grove State Hospital in Maryland, the question of the fear of death began to be studied when one of the patients in this facility who was being treated with LSD for his alcoholism recommended taking LSD to a nurse who had just been diagnosed with cancer. After the nurse followed his advice, which proved beneficial, the medical researchers at the center decided to open a new line of research, exploring LSD's ability to reduce the existential distress associated with death. Simultaneously, Eric Kast, M.D. was also conducting some studies at the University of

Chicago. While studying the analgesic potential of LSD in terminally ill patients, he observed that, in addition to its analgesic effects, LSD also appeared to reduce the fear of death and improve the quality of sleep for some time following the psychedelic experience.

Twenty years after the prohibition of LSD and psilocybin, research on patients suffering from depression and anxiety due to cancer or other terminal illnesses was resumed by several laboratories using both LSD and psilocybin.

A study at the University of Bern, led by the Swiss psychiatrist Peter Gasser, M.D., found a significant reduction in anxiety that still persisted after twelve months. The treatment consisted of conventional psychotherapy sessions supplemented by two psychedelic sessions, separated by an interval of two to three weeks. Both sessions consisted of high doses of LSD (200 micrograms) together with three 60- to 90-minute integration sessions after each experimental session. Eight participants received these high doses, while four received a subperceptual dose of 20 micrograms. In a second phase, three of the latter four individuals who received the subperceptual dose also underwent two psychedelic sessions in which they received the two 200-microgram doses of LSD.

Other studies using high doses of psilocybin in somewhat larger samples have found similar results. One study led by Stephen Ross, M.D. at New York University, with about fifteen patients per experimental group, found that anxiety had more than halved in 84 percent of patients seven weeks after therapy assisted with a single high dose of psilocybin. In the control group, which received niacin (an active placebo capable of causing physical, but not psychological sensations), this was the case in only 14 percent of them. The reduction was six times greater in the psilocybin group! Similar effects were found for the reduction of depressive symptoms, with effects significantly persisting at the twenty-six-week mark.

Finally, another study led by Ronald Griffiths from Johns Hopkins University has also found beneficial and long-lasting effects after a single high dose of psilocybin coupled with conventional psychotherapy. In this study, there were about twenty-five patients per group (i.e., a total of fifty-one patients in the study). By the five-week mark, anxiety and depressive symptoms were at least halved in three times as many participants in the high-dose psilocybin group than in the control group. Again, the effects lasted for several months: after six months, 61 percent of the participants were still in remission from depression and anxiety!

The results thus far seem to suggest that, at least under these therapeutic conditions, the psychedelic experience has the potential to improve attitudes and feelings of dread associated with impending death.

Addictions—Psilocybin and Other Psychedelics

During the introduction, we already mentioned how the treatment of alcohol addiction was one of the first researched psychotherapeutic uses of LSD. In fact, the cofounder of Alcoholics Anonymous, Bill Wilson, used it to treat his alcoholism.

More recent studies have favored the use of psilocybin, partly because its effects last about half as long as those of LSD, and partly because the molecule psilocybin does not have the LSD-attached stigma. In addition to psilocybin, another very peculiar substance, ibogaine, is also being used within the addiction field. Having a different mechanism of action than classic psychedelics such as psilocybin, LSD, or DMT (the psychoactive component of ayahuasca), this substance seems to be able to help combat the dreadful addiction to opioids. Since it is not a classic psychedelic, we will not review clinical studies with ibogaine nor its mechanism of action, but it is worth briefly mentioning that ibogaine not only acts on opioid receptors but also blocks the massive release of dopamine induced by drugs of abuse. By doing so, it is apparently able to mitigate withdrawal symptoms not only at the psychological level but also at the physiological one. Hopefully, future publications will be able to focus more on this complex substance.

Returning to psilocybin, only two preliminary studies have been carried out so far to treat addictions. One focused on tobacco addiction and the one on alcohol addiction, and, although limited, the results seem promising.

Johns Hopkins University has once again been a pioneer, this time with a study led by Matthew Johnson investigating tobacco addiction.

In this study published in 2014, smoking at least ten cigarettes per day and having failed at several quit attempts were among the specific inclusion criteria.

The study lasted fifteen weeks during which a weekly session of cognitive behavioral therapy based on the *Quit for Life* smoking cessation program was applied. In addition, participants were accompanied during two psychedelic sessions. Twenty milligrams of psilocybin were administered in the first session, which occurred on the fifth week of the study. This was already a perceptible dose. The next psychedelic session was carried out two weeks later, and the dose was increased to 30 mg. Finally, at the thirteenth week, depending on the participant's preference, there was an optional third dose of either 20 mg or 30 mg. All but two participants accepted it.

The results revealed that after six months, 80 percent of participants in this study were still smoke-free. In a follow-up study, 67 percent were still smoke-free at twelve months, this being corroborated by biomarkers in urine samples. Additionally, between sixteen and fifty-seven months (at an average of thirty months), 80 percent of the study participants were urine tested again, and 60 percent remained abstinent.

Although the sample size was very small, consisting only of fifteen participants, abundant psychological support was received and a control group was lacking, such results were particularly remarkable for several reasons. On the one hand, according to Johnson, other smoking cessation methods (both biomedical and psychotherapeutic) have a maximum efficacy of 35 percent, i.e., much lower than that observed here. Moreover, the fifteen participants in this group had been smoking, on average, nineteen cigarettes a day for thirty years and had tried to quit smoking six times. Certainly, they were highly addicted! Thanks to these results, in October 2021, the U.S. government funded for the first time psychedelic-assisted therapy research. Let us hope that the next step will be to appropriately reclassify these molecules. This is long overdue.

The second study was carried out at the University of New Mexico by a group led by Rick Strassman and instead studied alcohol addiction. In this case, psychotherapists used motivational therapy, commonly used to treat addictions, on nine patients for twelve weeks. In addition, two psychedelic sessions using perceptible doses were conducted, one at the fourth and another at the eighth week. In the first four weeks of the study, where only motivational therapy was used, a reduction in consumption was already observed; however, it was significantly accentuated after the first psychedelic session. For thirty-six weeks following the first session, the researchers monitored alcohol consumption and compared the data with consumption the month before beginning treatment. They found a significant reduction in alcohol consumption, measured as total days of abstinence and total days with large alcohol consumption.

A very common question arises when talking about eliminating addiction to one substance by using another. Isn't there a risk of replacing one addiction, in this case to tobacco or alcohol, with an addiction to psilocybin? Although it is a logical question, the answer is that this is not the case. It is true that, as we feel the benefits of this experience dissipate, we are in danger of wanting to return to it in search of more answers and new rebirths without having first made the effort to apply the learned lessons on a daily basis. Yet, the psychedelic experience is not something that one craves. Not only is there no such anxious anticipation, as happens with tobacco, alcohol, heroin, or even sugar; it is even quite common to develop a repulsion toward it, particularly when it comes to ingesting something such as a plant or a mushroom. The psychedelic experience is not an easy one. As a result, one gains tremendous respect for the substance, having to rather force oneself to consume it.

Or at least that was my case. It happened in England, after drinking a 30-gram tea of the famous "liberty caps" (*Psilocybe semilanceata*), gathered from the fruitful English grasslands the previous day. I remember that first time, I had no trouble drinking the tea. It didn't even taste bad to me. It was quite a high dose, especially considering my light weight, and it didn't take long for it to hit me. It was a steep takeoff. Immediately, and I ignored for how long, I was transported to a tremendous peace. Silence. Nothingness. Until, all of a sudden, a strange voice appeared, suddenly pulling me out of wherever it was I had been.

What? What is this? Hello?

Hello.

Who are you?

I don't know.

Does it matter?

I don't know.

What do you want? Peace or the pursuit of answers?

I don't know.

I choose peace. Silence.

I? Who is "I?"

And after several hours of pondering these questions and decisions, the end result was a profound sense of connection with the whole of humankind. All of us plunged together into this question and this strange experience called consciousness.

As I "landed" I felt a certain determination to write to my mother, and as I did so something happened. Powerful and deep emotions erupted from the core of my being in what was a deep and cleansing cry. She thought I was euphoric, which is understandable, considering that I began the message by telling her that I had just returned from an incredible adventure at the hands of hallucinogenic mushrooms. Despite her concern, the truth is that it was a very pleasant, meaningful, and healing journey. Or at least that's how I perceived it. My body, however, didn't seem to feel the same way.

As I walked through the countryside a few days later, I was overcome with a tremendous revulsion when I smelled the characteristic autumnal fungal dampness. Although during the psychedelic trip, as far as I can remember, I did not experience nausea or any other kind of discomfort, since that day, the very idea of consuming mushrooms (even a microdose!) gives me a strong feeling of disgust. Clearly, my body has learned a lesson: not to play with this magic substance. Although this rejection is not felt by everyone, nor is it as frequent when ingesting molecules such as LSD that have been synthesized in the laboratory, this bodily reaction is certainly a notable deterrent to developing an addictive behavior. But this is not the only reason why psychedelics are not addictive. Through mechanisms that we will study further on, these substances can help us find the determination needed to change addictive behaviors and other bad habits in our lives.

Obsessive-Compulsive Disorder (OCD)—Psilocybin

The line of research focused on the application of psychedelic therapy to treat obsessive-compulsive disorder (OCD) is even less conclusive than that of the other psychopathologies, but it is still worth mentioning briefly.

This disorder is characterized by obsessive and intrusive thoughts that cause high levels of anxiety. In an effort to reduce them, patients engage in repetitive and uncontrollable behaviors. Given the potential therapeutic effects of psychedelics on other psychopathologies that display symptoms also present in OCD (the intrusive thoughts of depression, the high anxiety linked to fear of death, or the uncontrolled behaviors of addictions), it would not be surprising if the symptoms of OCD could also be ameliorated after the psychedelic experience.

People with obsessive-compulsive disorder show a poor response to other available pharmacological treatments. In extreme cases, ablative[9] neurosurgery has had to be used to help combat the symptoms, so the limited results thus far obtained provide a window of hope, so far absent, for these patients.

To the best of my knowledge, there is only one experimental study carried out to treat obsessive-compulsive disorder. It was a preliminary study with only nine patients, led by Francisco Moreno at the University of Arizona in Tucson. During several sessions, separated by at least one week, increasing and detectable doses of psilocybin (100, 200, and 300 micrograms per kilogram) were administered. The evolution of symptoms was measured for twenty-four hours after each session and compared with the magnitude of symptoms at the beginning of each session.

In what was an interesting design, a fourth session with a superceptual dose (25 micrograms per kilogram) was included as a control. This session was randomly positioned somewhere between the other sessions, but never at the start. The study always began with the light but

---

9. This surgery involves destroying a piece of the brain.

noticeable 100-microgram dose. Surprisingly, the analyses showed that all sessions, even the subperceptual one, were able to reduce obsessive-compulsive symptoms. This triggers a cascade of questions.

Can we continue to use the subperceptual dose as a control in future studies? In the study in question, this subperceptual session always took place after having taken at least one noticeable dose of psilocybin; would the control dose have also been effective had it been administered before having had any previous psychedelic sessions, or can we perhaps attribute the effects observed in this control session to the expectation generated by the previous session and be solely a placebo effect?

In the placebo effect, bodily sensations and responses change in response to a thought, a sensation, or a wish fulfilled. They change in response to something immaterial, and not due to a pharmacological reason. In short, the placebo effect refers to the ability that mental dispositions have to affect bodily responses and their perception.

As we shall see, the psychedelic experience promotes the creation of new meanings as well as the transformation of old ones. Could it then be that, through its pharmacological changes, it acts, as Ido Hartogsohn at Harvard University suggests, as an enhancer of the placebo effect, making the person more suggestible to improving their symptoms by changing their map of meanings? Or, on the contrary, do the surprising results obtained with the control dose point to a possible pharmacological mechanism that is effective in OCD patients even with subperceptual doses? We do not know the answers to these questions, and what is more, they are not mutually exclusive. Moreover, we should not pay too much attention to the results of such a preliminary study. It is, however, worth mentioning that patients with obsessive-compulsive disorder tend to be considerably more resistant to the placebo effect than patients with other anxiety disorders, as a 2017 meta-analysis from the Hebrew University of Jerusalem led by Michael Sugarman showed. Perhaps the results observed in this study could go beyond a mere placebo effect. Perhaps they are simply the result of the therapeutic setting and the participants' expectations. Future research will have to answer all these questions.

MDMA-Assisted Therapy

Post-Traumatic Stress Disorder (PTSD)

Of all research lines focused on using psychoactive drugs during the psychotherapeutic process, this is undoubtedly the most advanced one. In fact, it is expected that by 2023 the FDA will finally grant MDMA medicinal status. Once this happens, doctors will be able to prescribe it, within a psychotherapeutic context, for the treatment of post-traumatic stress disorder (PTSD). As its name reveals, PTSD begins after a highly traumatic event. Studies have included, for example, war veterans, police officers, firefighters, victims of sexual abuse, or, more generally, people who have experienced a life-threatening event.

The enormous breakthrough in this line of clinical research would not have been possible without the work of the one and only Rick Doblin. His MAPS foundation has raised more than $100 million since prohibition. This money has mostly been used to fund a multitude of studies. From the first to the last, the results suggest that this new therapy is capable of alleviating suffering in a more effective way than any other therapy so far available. Thanks to these results, people who need it are closer than ever to having access to this treatment!

In the current psychedelic renaissance, the first study looking into MDMA's psychotherapeutic potential occurred between 2000 and 2002 and was led by José Carlos Bouso. It was a collaboration between MAPS, the Universidad Autónoma de Madrid, and the Universidad Autónoma de Barcelona. This study focused on researching MDMA-assisted therapy in twenty-nine victims of sexual abuse. However, despite being accepted by the Ministry of Health and an ethics committee, the government ended up banning its development due to media and political pressure. Data could only be obtained for six participants. These participants underwent three preparation sessions before the psychoactive session and three integration sessions afterward. Two of them received a placebo, three a 50-mg dose, and the remaining one a 75-mg dose. Although the small sample size precluded a valid statistical analysis, the results showed that the patient who received the 75 mg improved more than those who received the

50 mg, and those who received the 50 mg improved more than those who received the placebo.

The first study that could be fully carried out was published in 2010. In this study, led by Michael Mithoefer, the inclusion criterion was to be suffering from severe or moderate post-traumatic stress disorder and not to have improved neither after six months of psychotherapy nor after at least three months of conventional drug treatment.

Out of eighty-eight people willing to participate, only twenty-three made it through the selection process. For example, participants with bipolar or borderline personality disorder were not accepted. Once selected, and during the six weeks prior to the first dose of MDMA, two 90-minute preparation sessions were held with their designated psychotherapists. On the day of the MDMA intake, participants received 125 mg of MDMA (a high dose) and if they wished, after approximately two hours, they could receive another 62.5-mg dose. In total, the MDMA session lasted eight hours and the participants spent the night at the facility in order to have their first 90-minute integration session the following morning. During the following month, they underwent three more integration sessions (approximately one per week) before receiving a second MDMA session. Again, the second psychoactive session was followed by four integration sessions. Additionally, a daily telephone call was conducted during the week following each of the MDMA sessions. As you can see, it is not only a matter of offering MDMA but of offering this substance within an intensive psychotherapeutic process.

This study consisted of a total of twenty participants, twelve of whom received MDMA-assisted therapy, while the remaining eight received a placebo. The degree of post-traumatic stress disorder was measured at the beginning of the treatment and two months after completing it using a semi-structured interview. When the participants' characteristics were studied, they had been suffering from PTSD for an average of nineteen years. In addition, 75 percent of them had not only unsuccessfully completed more than one course of psychotherapy, but they had also tried an average of four different pharmacological treatments without obtaining any benefit. The results of this preliminary study were astonishing: while two months after the end of the study only 25 percent of the participants in the control group had responded to therapy, 83 percent of the participants in the MDMA group had responded!

After the end of the study, participants in the placebo group could receive MDMA-assisted therapy if they so wished. The active group also had the opportunity to receive a third MDMA session, coupled with the usual psychotherapeutic protocol.

Additionally, a follow-up of the participants' condition was carried out between seventeen and seventy-four months posttreatment. Only two participants had relapsed after this period of time. What was most striking was that an overall decline in the benefits obtained after MDMA-assisted therapy was not observed.

These excellent results prompted MAPS to carry out other similar studies in search of the optimal protocol. These studies vary somewhat. For example, in some cases, instead of receiving a placebo, the control group received a detectable dose of MDMA, either 25 mg or 40 mg. Although these are detectable doses, they don't seem to be high enough to offer significant therapeutic benefit, making them a good choice as an active placebo. When all these studies (a total of six) were included in a meta-analysis, the results were still encouraging, although not as striking as those from the first study. One of the reasons for this discrepancy may have been that, in some, the control group also received some MDMA. This meta-analysis included a total of seventy-two participants in the active group and thirty-one participants in the control group. After completing therapy assisted with two high doses of MDMA, 54 percent of the participants in the active group no longer had a diagnosis of post-traumatic stress disorder, compared to only 22.6 percent of the control group. Furthermore, when long-term follow-up was conducted after an average of 3.4 years, the results not only revealed that the benefits had not diminished over time; they also showed that they had continued to increase after the therapy had ended! This is probably because the treatment of trauma-related stress allowed other aspects regarding general well-being and interpersonal relationships to improve as well. In terms of negative side effects or harms caused by the therapy, only 8.3 percent reported having suffered some kind of harm, and of these, only 3.1 percent reported such harm persisting for over a year after the end of the therapy. Despite this, none of the participants considered it to be a serious harm and all reported benefitting from the therapy.

Thanks to these results, in August 2017, the FDA granted "breakthrough therapy" status to MDMA-assisted therapy for post-traumatic stress disorder. This allowed participants that had not received MDMA during the study (due to exclusion criteria or because they had belonged to the control group) to receive it outside the research setting. This is something that does not usually happen before molecules are granted medicinal status.

Finally, the last study published in 2021, led by Jennifer Mitchell, directly compared two groups of forty-five people. One group received three psychoactive sessions during MDMA-assisted therapy and the other, placebo-assisted therapy. Participants in both groups had gotten to know their psychotherapists gradually over approximately two months before the first experimental session (i.e., music with MDMA or placebo), having had a total of three 90-minute preparation sessions over those two months.

Before the last preparation session began, levels of post-traumatic stress were measured, in addition to the degree of disability and depression caused by the disorder. Participants were invited to take part in the first experimental session a few days later. Those in the MDMA group received 80 mg at the beginning of the session and, if they wished, a 40-mg booster approximately two hours later. Following the usual MDMA-assisted therapy protocol, they received a total of four integration sessions over the next month, before embarking on the second psychoactive session. The dose in this session was increased to 120 mg with an optional 60-mg booster. After this session, the previous integration process was repeated before the third psychoactive session. Both the dose of the second session and the integration process were repeated, there being a total of eighteen weeks between the first experimental session and the last integration session (figure 34). Two months after the end of the treatment, levels of post-traumatic stress, disability, and depression were again measured. Once again, the results were encouraging. While in the MDMA group, 33 percent of the participants were in remission at this time point, this was the case for only 5 percent of the control group. A huge difference! Furthermore, significant differences between the two groups were also observed in the reduction of disability and depressive symptoms.

The same as for depression, the most common psychotropic drugs used to treat post-traumatic stress disorder are SSRIs, specifically, sertraline and paroxetine. Unlike what has been done for depression, where the effectiveness of escitalopram was compared with that of psilocybin, no study has yet been carried out directly comparing MDMA-assisted therapy with SSRI-assisted therapy in patients with PTSD. However, several factors suggest that MDMA-assisted therapy is likely to be more effective. For one thing, 40 to 60 percent of patients with PTSD do not respond to SSRIs and prefer psychotherapy. However, the most effective psychotherapies applied for PTSD consist of patients having to confront and expose themselves to the traumatic memory. This is extremely painful and threatening, which is why the drop-out rate is particularly high for this population. A meta-analysis estimated an average of 29 percent drop-out rate. Meanwhile, in the meta-analysis conducted on MDMA studies, only 7.6 percent of the participants dropped out of this therapy.

The high efficacy observed across studies for MDMA-assisted therapy also appears to achieve higher levels of efficacy than those observed

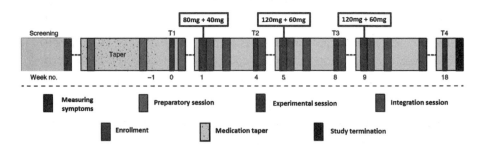

Figure 34. Diagram of the protocol used in Mitchell's MDMA-assisted therapy study. Image obtained from the study led by Mitchell, published in *Nature Medicine* in 2021. (See also color plate 13.)

for other therapies. Nevertheless, it will be necessary to carry out a study that directly compares the use of the psychotropic drug in question with that of MDMA within the same psychotherapeutic process. Only then will we be able to confirm, based on solid scientific evidence, the superiority of this molecule over other psychotropic drugs. That said, being aware of the particular psychoactive effects of MDMA, which we will see in later chapters, and in light of the results obtained so far, it will not be surprising if such supremacy is demonstrated in the coming years.

Alcohol Abuse

The use of MDMA-assisted therapy to treat substance abuse has been explored in two different studies.

One of these has been conducted with those participants with post-traumatic stress disorder in the latest study led by Mitchell. In an attempt to alleviate the distress caused by the disorder, these individuals often turn to substance use, with some studies estimating that between 17 percent and 46 percent of patients do so. Therefore, the study led by Mitchell included people who were currently showing, in addition to PTSD, a mild alcohol abuse disorder, as well as people who had been in remission from a moderate alcohol abuse disorder for the past three months. To assess the decrease in alcohol consumption, the level of alcohol consumption during the twelve months prior to treatment was assessed through questionnaires, and a significant decrease was found when comparing previous alcohol consumption with that of the two months after MDMA therapy. Although statistically significant, this decrease was not particularly large, nor was it correlated with a decrease in post-traumatic stress symptoms. However, the reduction in alcohol consumption was found to be correlated with initial levels of post-traumatic stress. Those starting from a more severe disorder showed a greater reduction. Moreover, only people with a mild substance use disorder were accepted. If people with a more severe substance use problem had been included in the sample, the reduction in alcohol consumption might have been greater, as there would have been a greater scope for reduction. Future studies will need to confirm whether or not this is the case.

The potential of MDMA-assisted therapy to treat alcoholism is also being studied in people with severe and prolonged alcohol use without post-traumatic stress disorder. In 2019, David Nutt's team first published some preliminary results, which included only four participants, from a study led by Ben Sessa. One of the participants had been abusing alcohol for ten years, another one for twenty years, and the remaining two for thirty years. In this case, the MDMA-assisted therapy consisted of two MDMA sessions (125 mg + 62.5 mg of reinforcement each) separated by approximately one month, in addition to ten psychotherapeutic sessions during which motivational therapy was applied. The treatment lasted for a total of eight weeks. When alcohol consumption was assessed nine months later, two of them had not consumed alcohol again and the other two had only consumed a low amount of alcohol once.

Although very few people were involved in this preliminary publication, the results are striking when one considers that they all had a long history of problematic alcohol use. Moreover, out of the four participants, three of them had failed in previous attempts to quit. This study also provides us with some direct statements from the participants. For example, the participant who had been abusing alcohol for twenty years said the following:

> Better than other treatments, including inpatient detox . . . I enjoyed every moment of it. Thrilled to be part of the study . . . I feel energised . . . The treatment has worked for me, done me a lot of good. I've got a lot of confidence out of it. I'm calmer . . . It's given me what I wanted; to be cured, to not have the cravings, to look at life differently. I'm not so angry at everything . . . Being under MDMA was beautiful. It showed me the real me; the me without alcohol.

The full study, consisting of a total of fourteen participants, was finally published in 2021 in the *Journal of Psychopharmacology*, showing that the average alcohol consumption rate dropped from 130.6 units of alcohol per week at baseline to zero inmediately after the

8-week MDMA-assisted detox course. As time progressed up until the nine-month post-treatment follow-up, only 21 percent of the subjects in the group were heavily drinking again (i.e., drinking more than fourteen units of alcohol per week).[10] This is a great improvement if we compare it to the best currently available treatments, where it is estimated that nine-months post treatment a total of 75 percent of participants are heavily drinking again.

Within the recreational context, MDMA use has been commonly associated with an emotional "comedown" on the days following intake (which lasts around three days). As we will see in the following chapters, MDMA produces a massive release of serotonin; hence, it has been theorized that the supposed comedown may be due to biological readjustments triggered by the release of serotonin. For example, the body might react to such a release by reducing the number of serotonin receptors available on postsynaptic membranes. Alternatively, it could be that, after detecting excessive amounts of serotonin, the body increases the production of enzymes responsible for biodegrading the neurotransmitter. Both cases would ultimately result in a decrease of the available serotonin in the days following the intake, thus negatively affecting the emotional state. However, to the best of my knowledge, currently, these are only theories and further research is needed.

To explore the question of the comedown, the study using MDMA for alcohol use disorder discussed above also tracked participants' mood during the week following the MDMA intake, not finding any fluctuations in mood during this time period.

The disparity between these preliminary results on mood and anecdotal reports on MDMA-related comedown could be due to many factors that will need to be explored further in the future. To begin with, Sessa's study could simply be failing to find a real comedown effect due to its small sample size, which could be strongly driven by individual differences in comedown susceptibility. Another possibility

---

10. Two of the participants in the sample received a second eight-week MDMA-assisted detox course during the study.

is that the comedown associated with recreational MDMA use may be due to factors other than MDMA, such as excessive alcohol consumption or the sleep deprivation that often surrounds its use. It could also be that those reporting an emotional comedown may have consumed higher doses than those used in the study. Alternatively, the benefits gained from the therapy might be counteracting the possible emotional comedown caused by MDMA.

Either way, these preliminary results slightly challenge the notion that an increase in mood due to MDMA must always be followed by a subsequent decrease. Perhaps, "what goes up must come down" does not apply here, being quite likely that sleep deprivation and alcohol consumption are playing a central role in the emotional comedown that is anecdotally associated with MDMA use. That said, the body naturally tends to self-regulate, so MDMA abuse probably produces unwanted changes in the nervous system. Although the results in the literature looking into MDMA's toxicity are ambiguous (it is difficult to find a sample of people who only consume MDMA, without also consuming other substances such as cannabis), and not all find the same results, some studies have found indications that repeated use of MDMA may damage the nervous system and negatively affect certain cognitive functions. Be that as it may, this molecule has been consumed in recreational settings for decades and, as a study published in 2010 led by Valerie Curran from University College London looking into the harms associated with different psychoactive substances has shown, MDMA appears to be much safer than many other recreational substances, including alcohol. However, unlike classic psychedelics, where the associated harms are only psychological or behavioral, excessive, irresponsible, or uninformed use of MDMA can result in death. It is of vital importance to provide harm reduction education and always test the purity of the substance. You can find all relevant information regarding the safe use of MDMA (and other substances) at Energy Control, a program born in Barcelona in 1997, focused on reducing the risks associated with drug use by providing society with harm-reduction information and a substance testing service.

Social Anxiety Linked to Autism

Autism refers to a broad range of conditions used to define those people who, although showing an enormous variety among them, tend to focus excessively on a particular interest and, since birth, have trouble processing and understanding typical social dynamics.[11] For example, by analyzing the gaze of babies, it is possible to detect from a very early age the presence or absence of this condition. Specifically, autistic babies seem to process people's faces following a different pattern than neurotypical babies, focusing, for example, less on people's gaze and more on objects.

High-functioning autistic people are often aware of their difficulty to communicate with others and establish interpersonal relationships, which can as a consequence lead to social anxiety. Furthermore, there is evidence that autistic people do not respond in the same way as neurotypical people to psychotropic drugs often used to treat social anxiety. Therefore, they have no effective treatment available to address this discomfort.

As we will see in later chapters, among other things, MDMA is capable of reducing the fear of social rejection; hence it could be a good candidate to treat social anxiety.

Based on this potential, Alicia L. Danforth from the Los Angeles Research Institute has explored the effects of MDMA on autistic people in two different studies. One studied their experiences after taking MDMA on their own (i.e., outside of a clinical trial), while the other consisted of a clinical trial involving MDMA-assisted therapy for autistic people who presented high levels of social anxiety.

In the former, one hundred autistic people completed online questionnaires related to the benefits achieved by using MDMA. The results showed that more than 70 percent reported feeling more comfortable in social situations, having an easier time communicating with others, or feeling more self-confident, after taking MDMA. Moreover, these effects persisted for at least a year.

---

11. The intensity of this impairment varies significantly from person to person, so it is more appropriate to refer to the "autistic spectrum" rather than to "autism."

Additionally, of those one hundred participants, twenty-four were invited to a semi-structured interview and, during the interview, 83 percent of them reported some significant positive change. For example, one of them said the following:

> I considered myself a machine in terms of emotions. I tried very hard not to succumb to any emotions. I felt that it was a stupid, a foolish human trait that I was above. And MDMA changed that.

Another commented on how, having been a hateful and depressed person for most of their life, they had become a loving one, as a result of experimenting with MDMA. And yet another one commented how even the person who accompanied them during the experience noted they had become a much happier and more confident person, as a result of the experience.

Finally, the textual words of another participant were as follows:

> . . . a lot of people that suffer mentally, you know, with self-image problems, and stuff like that would benefit immensely. Especially people with Asperger's, and you know autism spectrum, and people that have trouble vocalizing (their emotions).

It seems that MDMA was helping autistic people to feel a greater repertoire of emotions as well as improving their ability to socialize and communicate with others.

After finding these results, Danforth's next step was to conduct a pilot study offering MDMA-assisted therapy to autistic people suffering from high levels of social anxiety. A total of eleven people participated in this pilot study from 2018. Four were assigned to the control group, which received an inactive placebo during the psychotherapeutic process. The remaining seven had two sessions, one month apart, with MDMA. Following the usual MAPS protocol, there were three or four preparation sessions and three integration sessions during the month following each experimental session. After six months, social anxiety levels were measured in both groups and compared with baseline levels. Although the sample was very small, the results showed a greater, and statistically significant, reduction in those participants who had received MDMA-assisted therapy. These preliminary results seem to suggest that MDMA may alleviate the social anxiety that autistic individuals experience due to the confusion caused by having to navigate social norms that were not designed by and for them.

Naturally, these results lead to the following question: could MDMA, more generally, help people who, for reasons other than autism, suffer from social anxiety? This exciting (and likely) possibility will have to be explored soon, along with many others!

References for Further Study

Clinical Studies with Classic Psychedelics

Agin-Liebes GI, Malone T, Yalch MM, Mennenga SE, Ponté KL, Guss J, Bossis AP, Grigsby J, Fischer S, Ross S. 2020. Long-term follow-up of psilocybin-assisted psychotherapy for psychiatric and existential distress in patients with life-threatening cancer. Journal of Psychopharmacology 34(2):155–166.

Becker AM, Holze F, Grandinetti T, Klaiber A, Toedtli VE, Kolaczynska KE, Duthaler U, Varghese N, Eckert A, Grunblatt, et al. 2022. Acute effects of psilocybin after escitalopram or placebo pretreatment in a randomized, double-blind, placebo-controlled, crossover study in healthy subjects. Clinical Pharmacology & Therapeutics 111(4):886–895.

Bogenschutz MP, Forcehimes AA, Pommy JA, Wilcox CE, Barbosa PC, Strassman RJ. 2015. Psilocybin-assisted treatment for alcohol dependence: a proof-of-concept study. Journal of Psychopharmacology 29(3):289–299.

Carhart-Harris RL, Bolstridge M, Rucker J, Day CM, Erritzoe D, Kaelen M, Bloomfield M, Rickard JA, Forbes B, Feilding A, et al. 2016. Psilocybin with psychological support for treatment-resistant depression: an open-label feasibility study. The Lancet Psychiatry 3(7):619–627.

Carhart-Harris RL, Bolstridge M, Day CMJ, Rucker J, Watts R, Erritzoe DE, Kaelen M, Giribaldi B, Bloomfield M, Pilling S, et al. 2018. Psilocybin with psychological support for treatment-resistant depression: six-month follow-up. Psychopharmacology 235(2):399–408.

Carhart-Harris R, Giribaldi B, Watts R, Baker-Jones M, Murphy-Beiner A, Murphy R, Martell J, Blemings A, Erritzoe D, Nutt DJ. 2021. Trial of psilocybin versus escitalopram for depression. New England Journal of Medicine 384(15):1402–1411.

Davis AK, Barrett FS, May DG, Cosimano MP, Sepeda ND, Johnson MW, Finan PH, Griffiths RR. 2021. Effects of psilocybin-assisted therapy on major depressive disorder: a randomized clinical trial. JAMA Psychiatry 78(5):481–489.

Farzin D, Mansouri N. 2006. Antidepressant-like effect of harmane and other beta-carbolines in the mouse forced swim test. European Neuropsychopharmacology 16(5):324–328.

Fortunato JJ, Réus GZ, Kirsch TR, Stringari RB, Stertz L, Kapczinski F, Pinto JP, Hallak JE, Zuadri AW, Crippa, JA, et al. 2009. Acute harmine administration induces antidepressive-like effects and increases BDNF levels in the rat hippocampus. Progress in neuro-psychopharmacology & biological psychiatry 33(8):1425–1430.

Fortunato JJ, Réus GZ, Kirsch TR, Stringari RB, Fries GR, Kapczinski F, Hallak JE, Zuadri AW, Crippa, JA, Qeuevdo J. 2010. Chronic administration of harmine elicits antidepressant-like effects and increases BDNF levels in rat hippocampus. Journal of neural transmission (Vienna, Austria: 1996) 117(10):1131–1137.

Gasser P, Holstein D, Michel Y, Doblin R, Yazar-Klosinski B, Passie T, Brenneisen R. 2014. Safety and efficacy of lysergic acid diethylamide-assisted psychotherapy for anxiety associated with life-threatening diseases. The Journal of Nervous and Mental Disease 202(7):513.

Goodwin GM, Croal M, Feifel D, Kelly JR, Marwood L, Mistry S, O'Keane V, Peck SK, Simmons H, Sisa C, et al. 2023. Psilocybin for treatment resistant depression in patients taking a concomitant SSRI medication. Neuropsychopharmacology 48(10):1492–1499.

Goodwin GM, Aaronson ST, Alvarez O, Atli M, Bennett JC, Croal M, DeBattista C, Dunlop BW, Feifel D, Hellerstein DJ, et al. 2023. Single-dose psilocybin for a treatment-resistant episode of major depression: impact on patient-reported depression severity, anxiety, function, and quality of life. Journal of affective disorders 327:120–127.

Griffiths RR, Johnson MW, Carducci MA, Umbricht A, Richards WA, Richards BD, Cosimano MP, Klinedinst MA. 2016. Psilocybin produces substantial and sustained decreases in depression and anxiety in patients with life-threatening cancer: a randomized double-blind trial. Journal of Psychopharmacology 30(12):1181–1197.

Grob CS, Danforth AL, Chopra GS, Hagerty M, McKay CR, Halberstadt AL, Greer GR. 2011. Pilot study of psilocybin treatment for anxiety in patients with advanced-stage cancer. Archives of General Psychiatry 68(1):71–78.

Krediet E, Bostoen T, Breeksema J, Van Schagen A, Passie T, Vermetten E. 2020. Reviewing the potential of psychedelics for the treatment of PTSD. International Journal of Neuropsychopharmacology 23(6):385–400.

Johnson MW, Garcia-Romeu A, Cosimano MP, Griffiths RR. 2014. Pilot study of the 5-HT2AR agonist psilocybin in the treatment of tobacco addiction. Journal of Psychopharmacology 28(11):983–992.

Johnson MW, Garcia-Romeu A, Griffiths RR. 2017. Long-term follow-up of psilocybin-facilitated smoking cessation. The American Journal of Drug and Alcohol Abuse 43(1):55–60.

Moreno FA, Wiegand CB, Taitano EK, Delgado PL. 2006. Safety, tolerability, and efficacy of psilocybin in 9 patients with obsessive-compulsive disorder. The Journal of Clinical Psychiatry 67(11):1735–1740.

Morales-García JA, de la Fuente Revenga M, Alonso-Gil S, Rodríguez-Franco M I, Feilding A, Perez-Castillo A, Riba J. 2017. The alkaloids of Banisteriopsis caapi, the plant source of the Amazonian hallucinogen Ayahuasca, stimulate adult neurogenesis in vitro. Scientific reports 7(1):5309.

Nutt DJ, King LA, Phillips LD. 2010. Drug harms in the UK: a multicriteria decision analysis. The Lancet 376(9752):1558–1565.

Osório FDL, Sanches RF, Macedo LR, Dos Santos RG, Maia-de-Oliveira JP, Wichert-Ana L, de Araujo DB, Riba J, Crippa JA, Hallak JE. 2015. Antidepressant effects of a single dose of ayahuasca in patients with recurrent depression: a preliminary report. Brazilian Journal of Psychiatry 37:13–20.

Ross S, Bossis A, Guss J, Agin-Liebes G, Malone T, Cohen B, Mennenga SE, Belser A, Kalliontzi K, Babb J, et al. 2016. Rapid and sustained symptom reduction following psilocybin treatment for anxiety and depression in patients with life-threatening cancer: a randomized controlled trial. Journal of Psychopharmacology 30(12):1165–1180.

Studerus E, Kometer M, Hasler F, Vollenweider FX. 2011. Acute, subacute and long-term subjective effects of psilocybin in healthy humans: a pooled analysis of experimental studies. Journal of Psychopharmacology 25(11):1434–1452.

Clinical Studies with MDMA

Danforth AL, Struble CM, Yazar-Klosinski B, Grob CS, Danforth AL. 2015. MDMA-assisted therapy: a new treatment paradigm for autistic adults with social anxiety. Progress in Neuropsychopharmacology & Biological Psychiatry doi: 10.1016/j.pnpbp.2015.03.011.

Danforth AL, Grob CS, Struble C, Feduccia AA, Walker N, Jerome L, Yazar-Klosinski B, Emerson A. 2018. Reduction in social anxiety after MDMA-assisted psychotherapy with autistic adults: a randomized, double-blind, placebo-controlled pilot study. Psychopharmacology 235(11):3137–3148.

Danforth AL. 2019. Embracing neurodiversity in psychedelic science: a mixed-methods inquiry into the MDMA experiences of autistic adults. Journal of Psychoactive Drugs 51(2):146–154.

Jerome L, Feduccia AA, Wang JB, Hamilton S, Yazar-Klosinski B, Emerson A, Mithoefer MC, Doblin R. 2020. Long-term follow-up outcomes of MDMA-assisted psychotherapy for treatment of PTSD: a longitudinal pooled analysis of six phase 2 trials. Psychopharmacology 237(8):2485–2497.

Mitchell JM, Bogenschutz M, Lilienstein A, Harrison C, Kleiman S, Parker-Guilbert K, Ot'alora GM, Garas W, Paleos C, Gorman I, et al. 2021. MDMA-assisted therapy for severe PTSD: a randomized, double-blind, placebo-controlled phase 3 study. Nature Medicine 27(6):1025–1033.

Mithoefer A, Jerome L, Ruse J, Doblin R, Gibson E, Marcela Ot'alora G M. 2013. A manual for MDMA-assisted psychotherapy in the treatment of posttraumatic stress disorder. Published by MAPS (Multidisciplinary Association of Psychedelics Studies).

Mithoefer MC, Wagner MT, Mithoefer AT, Jerome L, Doblin R. 2011. The safety and efficacy of ±3,4-methylenedioxymethamphetamine-assisted psychotherapy in subjects with chronic, treatment-resistant posttraumatic stress disorder: the first randomized controlled pilot study. Journal of Psychopharmacology 25(4):439–452.

Mithoefer MC, Feduccia AA, Jerome L, Mithoefer A, Wagner M, Walsh Z, Hamilton S, Yazar-Klosinski B, Emerson A, Doblin R. 2019. MDMA-assisted psychotherapy for treatment of PTSD: study design and rationale for phase 3 trials based on pooled analysis of six phase 2 randomized controlled trials. Psychopharmacology 236(9):2735–2745.

Sessa B, Sakal C, O'Brien S, Nutt D. 2019. First study of safety and tolerability of 3,4-methylenedioxymethamphetamine (MDMA)-assisted psychotherapy in patients with alcohol use disorder: preliminary data on the first four participants. BMJ Case Reports CP 12(7):e230109.

Sessa B, Higbed L, O'Brien S, Durant C, Sakal C, Titheradge D, Williams TM, Rose-Morris Anna, Brew-Girard E, Burrows S, et al. 2021. First study of safety and tolerability of 3,4-methylenedioxymethamphetamine-assisted psychotherapy in patients with alcohol use disorder. Journal of Psychopharmacology 35(4): 375–383.

3

Within the Psychedelic Experience

Before starting this rather long chapter, please note that we will dive deeply into the literature surrounding neuroimaging studies. As we advance, references will be made to studies mentioned earlier in the chapter. Although I have tried to always include all the information required for a good understanding, at the end of this chapter you will find summary tables of the different neuroimaging studies mentioned throughout its pages. The studies in the tables are organized according to different types of psychedelic effects. Thus, whenever you wish, you will be able to have a global and orderly overview of the different conditions under which the studies were carried out and the results associated with each one of them. Do also bear in mind that, although I have presented the phenomenological aspects of the psychedelic experience separately, it is most likely that they are all interrelated. After all, although some degree of functional segregation exists, the brain is a single interconnected network. As you will see, I have not dared to establish a clear hierarchy between them, and as I warned you at the beginning of the book, we will be faced with more questions than answers. With that being said, let's get started!

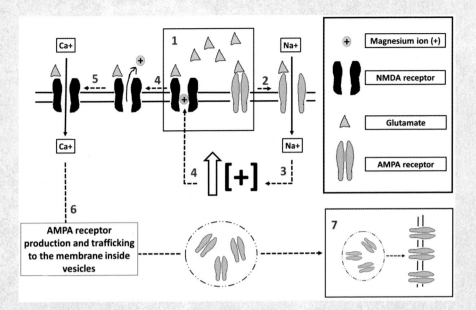

Plate 1. Mechanism of neuroplasticity through which a glutamatergic synapse in the cortex is strengthened. Step 1, glutamate binds to NMDA receptor and AMPA; step 2, activation of AMPA; step 3, increase in positive charge inside the neuron through AMPA; step 4, positive charge in the interior of the neuron reaches a threshold that repels the magnesium ion unblocking the NMDA receptor; step 5, massive calcium influx; step 6, intracellular signaling; and step 7, insertion of AMPA receptors into the membrane.

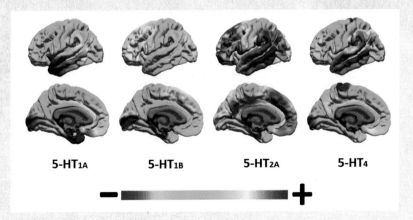

Plate 2. Distribution maps of four types of serotonin (5-HT) receptors: two from family 1, one from family 2, and one from family 4. In red, the areas with a high density of the corresponding receptor can be seen, and in blue the areas with a lower density. Image obtained from a study led by Beliveau et al and published in *The Journal of Neuroscience* in 2017.

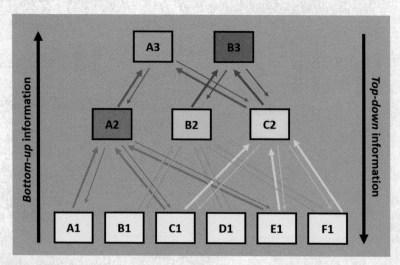

Plate 3. Diagram of the convergence of information. In this diagram, neuron A2, placed at the second level of integration is receiving information from the first-order neurons A1, C1, and E1, while the second-order neuron B2 is receiving information from the first-order neurons B1, D1, and F1. Equally, neuron C2 is receiving information from C1, E1, and F1. When neuron A2 fires an action potential to the corresponding third-order neuron (A3), it will transmit integrated information from A1, C1, and E1, while neuron B2 will transmit integrated information from B1, D1, and F1. And in the same way, information from second-order neurons will converge on third-order ones. Regulatory information (i.e., top-down information from higher to lower levels) is also shown.

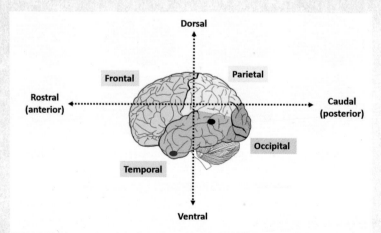

Plate 4. Illustration of the cerebral lobes. Each color represents a brain lobe. The different orientations of the brain are also shown, which apply to all brain lobes (e.g., the red dot is located in the anteroventral temporal lobe and the black dot in the posterodorsal temporal lobe).

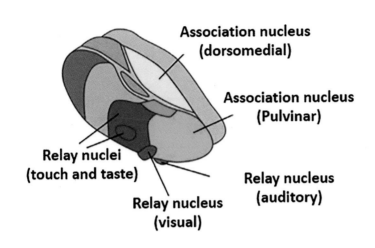

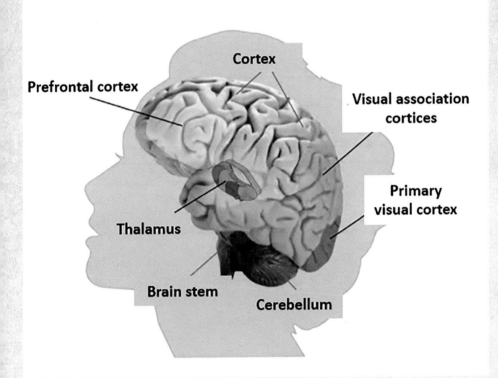

Plate 5. A schematic representation of some thalamic nuclei (*above*) and their corresponding cortical projections (*below*), represented through the matching colors. Image by Nadal and Amarillo, 2018, published in *Science Today*.

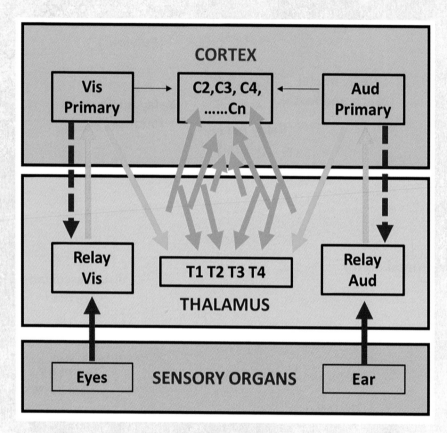

Plate 6. The orange box at the *bottom* represents the sensory organs. The blue one in the *middle* represents the thalamus and the green one *above* the cortex. T1, T2, T3, T4: association thalamic nuclei; C2, C3, C4 . . . Cn: heteromodal and associative cortices; Aud: auditory; Vis: visual.

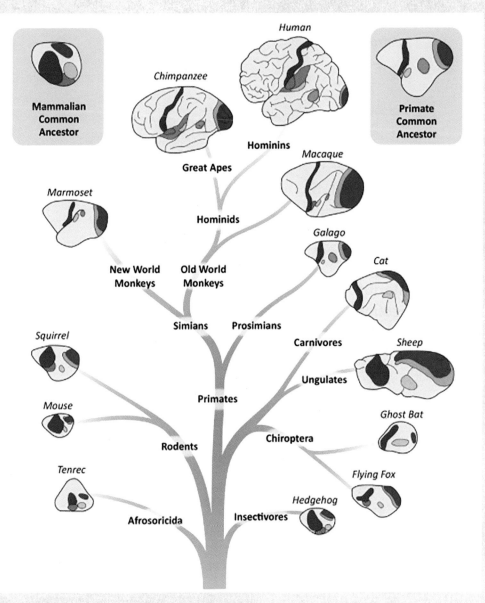

Plate 7. Phylogenetic tree of the brain. The colored areas show the different primary cortices, whereas the association cortices are shown in gray. Image obtained from an article by Buckner and Krienen published in *Trends in Cognitive Sciences* in 2013.

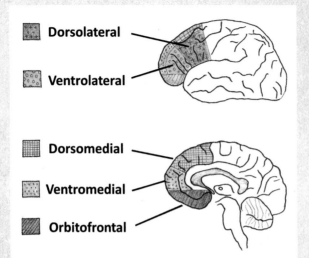

Plate 8. Subdivisions of the prefrontal cortex. A lateral plane of the brain is shown *above* and a medial plane *below*.

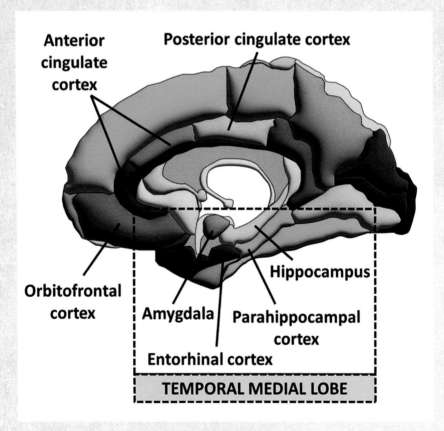

Plate 9. Visual representation of the cortical areas of the medial temporal lobe. Note their proximity to the hippocampus.

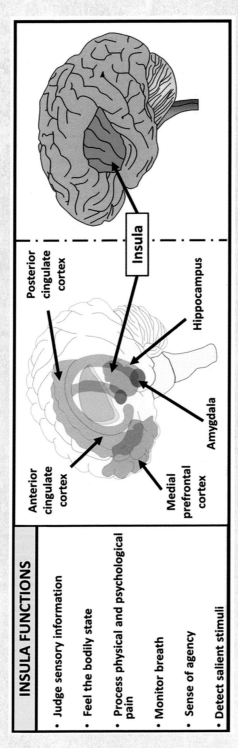

INSULA FUNCTIONS

- Judge sensory information
- Feel the bodily state
- Process physical and psychological pain
- Monitor breath
- Sense of agency
- Detect salient stimuli

Anterior cingulate cortex

Posterior cingulate cortex

Medial prefrontal cortex

Amygdala

Hippocampus

Insula

Plate 10. Functions and location of the insula. The first image shows the location of the insula in relation to the amygdala, and the second shows a more realistic representation of its location within the cortex, which is buried beneath the temporal and frontal cortex.

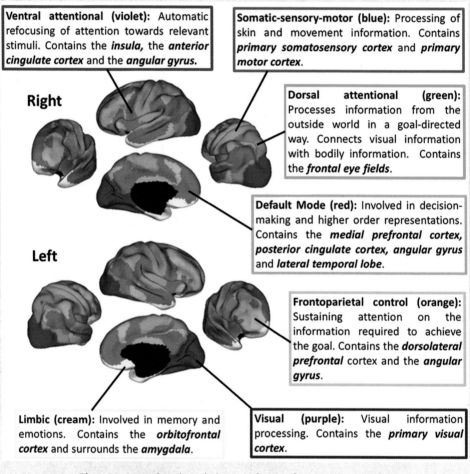

Ventral attentional (violet): Automatic refocusing of attention towards relevant stimuli. Contains the *insula,* the *anterior cingulate cortex* and the *angular gyrus.*

Somatic-sensory-motor (blue): Processing of skin and movement information. Contains *primary somatosensory cortex* and *primary motor cortex.*

Right

Dorsal attentional (green): Processes information from the outside world in a goal-directed way. Connects visual information with bodily information. Contains the *frontal eye fields.*

Default Mode (red): Involved in decision-making and higher order representations. Contains the *medial prefrontal cortex, posterior cingulate cortex, angular gyrus* and *lateral temporal lobe.*

Left

Frontoparietal control (orange): Sustaining attention on the information required to achieve the goal. Contains the *dorsolateral prefrontal* cortex and the *angular gyrus.*

Limbic (cream): Involved in memory and emotions. Contains the *orbitofrontal cortex* and surrounds the *amygdala.*

Visual (purple): Visual information processing. Contains the *primary visual cortex.*

Plate 11. Lateral and medial view of Yeo's functional networks.

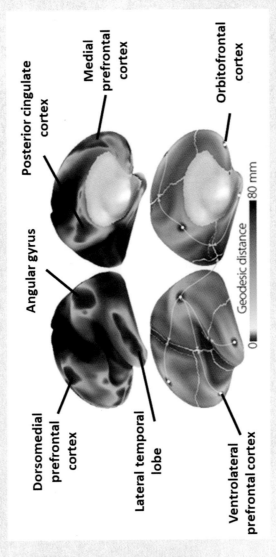

Posterior cingulate cortex

Medial prefrontal cortex

Orbitofrontal cortex

Angular gyrus

Dorsomedial prefrontal cortex

Lateral temporal lobe

Ventrolateral prefrontal cortex

Geodesic distance

0   80 mm

Plate 12. Gradient from the primary cortices (shown in blue) to the higher-order integration regions belonging to the default mode network (shown in red). Image obtained from a study led by Margulies et al. and published in *Proceedings of the National Academy of Sciences USA* in 2016.

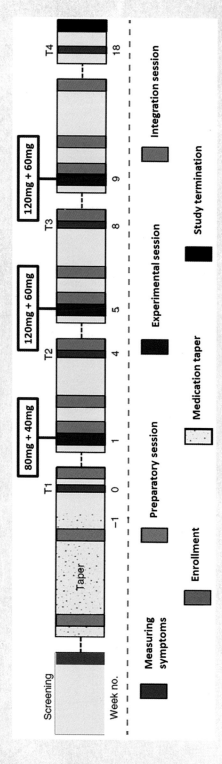

Plate 13. Diagram of the protocol used in Mitchell's MDMA-assisted therapy study. Image obtained from the study led by Mitchell, published in *Nature Medicine* in 2021.

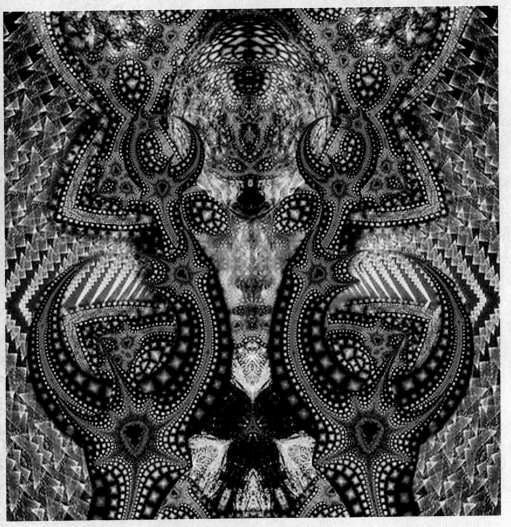

Plate 14. *Galactus Metal* by Bill Brouard.

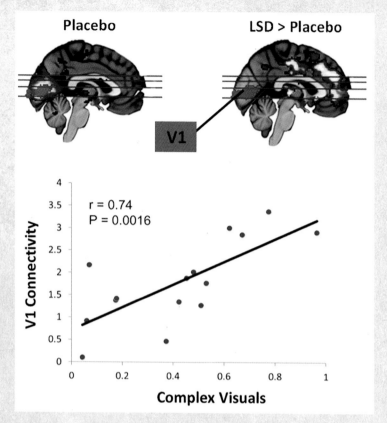

Plate 15. Connectivity changes in the primary visual cortex (V1). Image modified and obtained from Carhart-Harris et al., 2016, and published in *Proceedings of the National Academy of Sciences USA*.

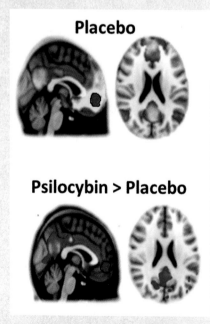

Plate 16. Changes in medial prefrontal cortex connectivity (red spot with black border). The top row shows the connectivity map during the placebo. The bottom row shows a subtraction of the map obtained with placebo and the map obtained with psilocybin (psilocybin > placebo), showing the specific changes in the connectivity map of this prefrontal area due to psychedelics. The blue color indicates areas with which the medial prefrontal cortex loses connectivity. Image taken from Carhart-Harris et al., published in *Frontiers in Human Neuroscience* in 2014.

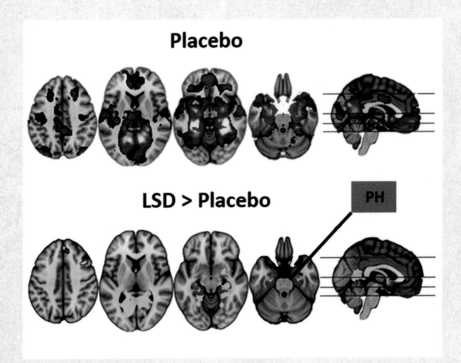

Plate 17. Changes in the connectivity map of the parahippocampal cortex (PH: shown in purple). The *top* row shows the connectivity map during the placebo. The *bottom* row shows a subtraction of the map obtained with the placebo and the map obtained with psilocybin, showing the specific changes in the connectivity of this limbic area due to LSD. Blue indicates areas with which it loses connectivity. Image obtained from Carhart-Harris et al., 2016, and published in *Proceedings of the National Academy of Sciences USA*.

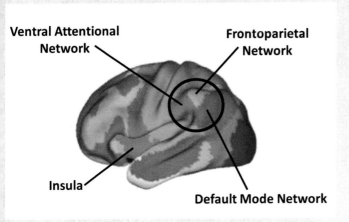

Plate 18. Image of the Yeo networks showing the convergence between various high-order networks in the angular gyrus (marked by the circle). The location of the insular cortex is also shown. Image modified from a study led by Yeo and published in the *Journal of Neurophysiology* in 2011.

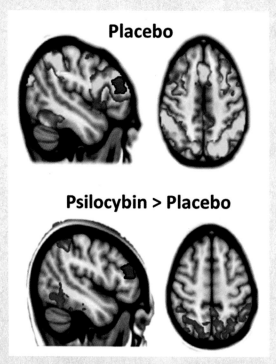

Placebo

Psilocybin > Placebo

Plate 19. Changes in the connectivity map of a central component of the frontoparietal executive network: the dorsolateral prefrontal cortex (red spot with black border). Its usual connectivity map is shown at the *top*. At the *bottom*, its changes under psilocybin. Blue shows areas with reduced connectivity to the dorsolateral prefrontal cortex under psilocybin. Image obtained from Carhart-Harris et al., published in *Frontiers in Human Neuroscience* in 2014.

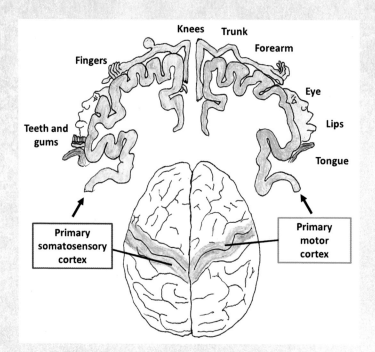

Plate 20. Penfield's homunculus of the somatic-sensory-motor cortex, showing in which areas of the cortex information from different parts of the body is represented (only some parts of the body are named).

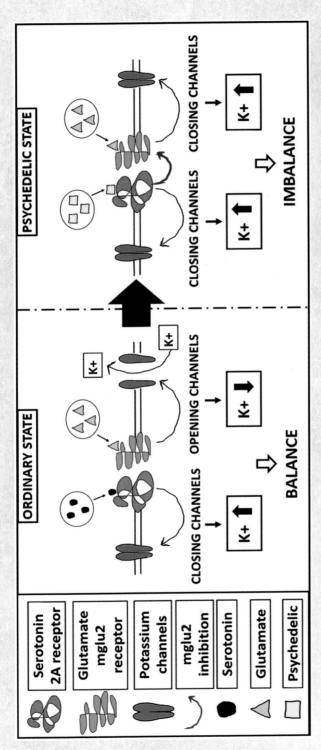

Plate 21. Function of the 2A-mglu2 heterodimer in ordinary states and under the action of a psychedelic. When, instead of serotonin, a psychedelic molecule binds to the 2A receptor, it inhibits the action of mglu2 (red arrow), producing an excessive accumulation of potassium in the interior of the neuron that causes a strong imbalance of charges, causing the spontaneous generation of action potentials.

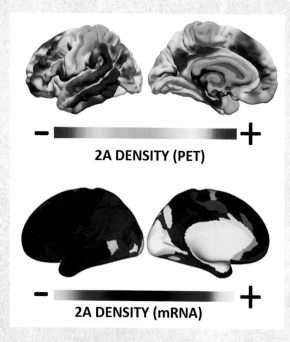

2A DENSITY (PET)

2A DENSITY (mRNA)

Plate 22. Serotonin 2A receptor distribution. *Above* is the distribution map of the 2A receptor using PET and *below* is the distribution map using messenger RNA (mRNA). The image *above* is modified from a study led by Beliveau and published in *The Journal of Neuroscience* in 2016. The *bottom* image was modified from a study led by Preller published in eLife in 2018.

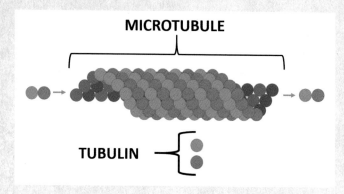

MICROTUBULE

TUBULIN

Plate 23. Diagram of a microtubule formed by tubulin proteins. Image obtained and modified from Simon Caulton.

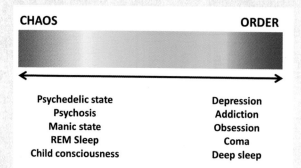

CHAOS   **ORDER**

Psychedelic state	Depression
Psychosis	Addiction
Manic state	Obsession
REM Sleep	Coma
Child consciousness	Deep sleep

Plate 24. The gradient between chaos and order in which the state of consciousness can be situated. Image modified from the article *The Entropic Brain* by Carhart-Harris et al., published in *Frontiers in Human Neuroscience* in 2014.

How can the effects of a single molecule transform, in such a significant way in such a short period of time, people who have been suffering from a series of clinical symptoms for years? How do these molecules transform the state of consciousness, and why can such transformation be therapeutic for the individual?

The Mystical Experience

Before taking a deep look into the different subjective effects present in the psychedelic experience and their relationship to changes in brain behavior, we should mention how these substances are capable of promoting a very particular experience: the mystical experience. Although such an experience can occur occasionally through certain practices, as well as emerge during a type of epileptic seizure originated in the medial temporal lobe, psychedelics have a particular capacity to promote it, and studies have repeatedly shown that the improvement in clinical symptoms is related to the intensity of this experience. What does this experience consist of? One of its characteristics is the impossibility of expressing it through language, but we will try anyway.

During the mystical experience, there is an absolute dissolution of the self, a dissolution that is accompanied by an ineffable sense of connection to the "whole." It is the hippies' classic statement that "we are one." And, in the face of this "whole," there is a feeling of reverence and deep gratitude. An appreciation for every being on earth, each one of them vibrant with life and consciousness.

The past and the future lose both their significance and their relevance. A wild prominence is, instead, given to the information contained in the experience of the present moment, from which a tremendous and previously ignored beauty now emerges along with feelings of incommensurable dimensions.

Awe, ecstasy, or the peace of the Buddha pervades your entire being and this new reality, now based on the present moment and the "oneness" of Nature, is perceived as more real than the previous one based on categories and mental narratives. The dreaded fleetingness of life, suddenly understood as an intrinsic part of the revered process that enables existence, is not only accepted but also embraced, as one perceives that there is something beyond matter, something greater than ourselves, that does remain beyond death. This is, of course, particularly beneficial for patients with depression and anxiety linked to terminal illness as shown by the correlations found between the improvement of symptoms and the intensity of the spiritual component experienced during the psychedelic session. But such a correlation is also present in studies on addiction and depression. It seems that the therapeutic potential of these substances goes beyond their pharmacological effects, being rather the result of that which one experiences during the altered state of consciousness.

In his article entitled *Becoming Gaia While Finding Myself,* Nick// Green Lantern, an Erowid[1] member, defines his mystical experience as follows:

> Amidst the breathtaking view of the horizon, in which I clearly saw every ripple in the ocean water, geometric hallucination in the sky, and mystic images of god-like faces, all accented to the hundredth power by the suns' heavenly rays, was a complete understanding of Gaia and its legacy. I realized with the [utmost] clarity, that everything on this earth; every human, every blade of grass, even every insipid pop-culture magazine, is a manifestation of the universe and serves as a vehicle of communication. My sense of identity had completely disappeared, as I was convinced with every fibre of my being that I was Gaia. As the sun set, I felt that I had transcended into a dimension far beyond what I knew to be the physical world.

Taken in high doses, the psychedelic experience is extremely powerful and intense. It can even be overwhelming. Our way of feeling and thinking abruptly changes, such a break with our ordinary state being perceived as a journey through the inner space of consciousness. No wonder this happens since there are changes of all sorts: perceptual, semantic, executive, emotional . . . Let's take a look at them!

---

1. Erowid is a nonprofit organization providing information and education on psychoactive substances. Their website can be found online.

Phenomenology and Neuroimaging

Visual Effects

Before the psychiatrist Humphry Osmond coined the term "psychedelic," these substances were commonly known as hallucinogens because of their ability to alter the perception of one's surroundings. However, if we consider hallucinations as "seeing something where there is nothing," this term is not correct, since this is not their real effect. Don't expect to see a flying dinosaur, at least not with your eyes open! Nope. More precisely, rather than hallucinations per se, these molecules cause visual distortions. The environment takes on a more unstable and changing quality. It can seem as if the objects around us have a certain pulse as if they are breathing, and sometimes, even the structure that makes up the three-dimensional space seems visible.

If you have never tried psychedelics this is impossible to conceive. Although there is not any nonpharmacological method capable of producing such visual effects, in the following QR code you can access a video that causes an optical illusion that, in my opinion, captures some aspects of such visual distortions. When you open the video, keep your eyes on the central point of the screen until it finishes. Then, look around you. To maximize the optical effect, I recommend that you do not look at a white wall, but at spaces containing certain complexity of edges and colors. Amazing, isn't it? As the video says: "We don't live in a world of reality but in a world of perception."

Scan the QR code to see an example of a visual distortion.

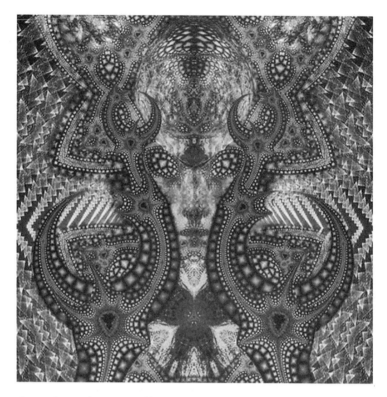

Figure 35. *Galactus Metal* by Bill Brouard. (See also color plate 14.)

That said, psychedelics can indeed promote hallucinations with closed eyes, but we refer to them as "visuals." Some of these visuals are scenes packed with geometric shapes, symmetry, fractals, or, as Albert Hofmann defined them after that first historic LSD trip, "kaleidoscopic." Visuals of a more complex nature full of symbolism can also be present. Entities, landscapes, architectural figures . . . and, as we shall see later, autobiographical elements often appear too. These visuals can be of such a magnitude that some people claim to have had to open their eyes in order to "stop seeing."

It is fascinating to study how there is a certain archetypal quality[2] in this symbolic material, as David Luke does. Luke is a psychologist

2. An archetype refers to the original pattern, model or prototype from which other objects, ideas, or concepts are derived.

particularly focused on investigating the phenomena of an apparently paranormal nature that is often present during altered states of consciousness. He is also the founder and director of the pioneering psychedelic conference "Breaking Convention" held in London every two years. When one studies, for example, the phenomenology described by users of vaporized DMT (the psychoactive principle in ayahuasca), it is very common for insect- or faunal-shaped entities to appear. These are perceived as intelligent, and there is more to it than the perception of sharing a physical space with them. A feeling of being able to communicate with them is also present. Terence McKenna, an American mystical ethnobotanist in the 1990s who advocated for the responsible use of psychedelics, called these entities "mechanical elves," a name that is still in use today. Multiple "psychonaut" artists have depicted them in spectacular and detailed works of art. In figure 35 or color plate 14, for example, you can see a piece called *Galactus Metal* by artist Bill Brouard. Amazing, isn't it?

For such visuals to occur, something must, logically, be occurring at the visual cortex, but, what exactly? What do neuroimaging studies find when they explore the behavior of this brain region during the psychedelic experience? One might, perhaps, expect to find an increased activity, but this is not the case. It seems that the secret does not lie within the activity levels of the visual cortex, but in other aspects such as its connectivity, as shown, for example, in color plate 15.[3] This image shows the result from a study in 2016 led by Carhart-Harris using functional magnetic resonance imaging. In this study, the connectivity of the primary visual cortex (V1, shown in pink in color plate 15) under the effects of a placebo was compared to that under the effects of LSD, while participants rested with their eyes closed inside the scanner. In the brain depicted on the left of color plate 15, you can see the connectivity map associated with V1 during

---

3. Image modified from the following article: Carhart-Harris RL, Muthukumaraswamy S, Roseman L, Kaelen M, Droog W, Murphy K, Tagliazucchi E, Schenberg EE, Nest T, Orban C, et al. 2016. Neural correlates of the LSD experience revealed by multimodal neuroimaging. Proceedings of the National Academy of Sciences USA 113(17):4853–4858.

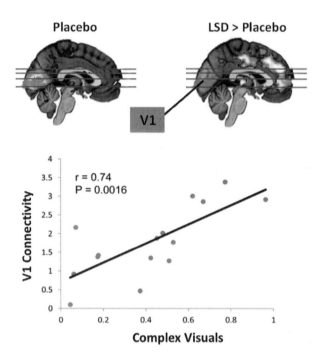

Figure 36. Connectivity changes in the primary visual cortex (V1). Image modified and obtained from Carhart-Harris et al., 2016, and published in *Proceedings of the National Academy of Sciences USA*. (See also color plate 15.)

the placebo condition. In this case, the connectivity map is limited to the occipital lobe. On the right, you can see the difference between the map obtained under LSD and the map obtained under the placebo (LSD>Placebo), showing how, during the psychedelic experience, the connectivity map of the primary visual cortex seems to extend toward associative areas with which it does not normally communicate, at least not during resting states.

In short, it seems that, during the psychedelic experience, signals from the visual cortex gain territory, expanding into areas involved in a higher order of integration. And guess what else! The degree of that expansion correlates with the intensity of complex visuals reported by participants: the greater V1's connectivity with the rest of the brain, the greater the complex visuals' intensity (see graph in color plate 15).

Let's consider how this might relate to the bottom-up and top-down information we discussed in chapter 1 when looking at how the brain integrates information.[4] Could the pattern of activity observed in this study be reflecting the ascent of signals from the visual cortex to associative areas? When we are at rest during ordinary states of consciousness, regulatory information (i.e., information travelling from higher levels to lower levels of integration) predominates over ascending information, but this changes when the system receives stimulation from the outside world. Hence, could the observed dominance of visual signals in associative areas be indicating that, when we close our eyes during the psychedelic experience, the brain behaves similarly to how it does when it is being visually stimulated? Since the method applied to study changes in the functional connectivity of the primary visual cortex under LSD using fMRI only allowed the establishment of a correlation between signals from different areas, but not a directionality, researchers at Imperial College London conducted a second study. This study used intravenous DMT and was led by Andrea Alamia and Christopher Timmermann. In addition, this time they used EEG, a technique that, as we saw in chapter 1, has a much higher temporal resolution than functional MRI.

The results of this study seemed to confirm the hypothesis: during the psychedelic experience, the electrical current travelled from electrodes located in the lower order areas related to visual processing to electrodes located in associative areas (figure 37[5]). Indeed, the pattern of brainwave directionality observed during the psychedelic experience was very similar to that observed when the brain is visually stimulated during ordinary states of consciousness. Moreover, the change in the ratio of upward to downward information was, again, highly correlated with the participants' subjective visual effects: the more upward currents predominated over downward ones, the

---

4. See figure 7 or the arrows traveling left down the deep cortical layers of figure 14 in chapter 1.
5. Image modified from the following article: Alamia A, Timmermann C, Nutt DJ, VanRullen R, Carhart-Harris RL. 2020. DMT alters cortical travelling waves. Elife 9:e59784.

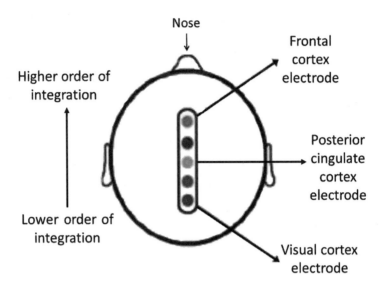

Figure 37. Position of EEG sensors (i.e., electrodes) on the head going from lower-order areas to higher-order areas of integration. Image modified from the study by Alamia et al., 2020, published in eLife.

bigger the subjective effects. Recall figure 14 from chapter 1. This would translate into an increase in the number of arrows pointing to the right and a decrease in the number of arrows pointing to the left.

In conclusion, it appears that, during the psychedelic experience, some aspects of the brain's behavior, even when our eyes are shut, resemble those occurring when the brain is processing visual information during ordinary states of consciousness, allowing us to imagine vivid fantastical images capable of undoubtedly capturing our full attention.

Using this same data set researchers also found a significant increase in the complexity of brain signals, meaning that signals became more chaotic and unpredictable during the psychedelic state. The greatest increases were found in the signals picked up from the electrodes from the visual cortex, and the change in complexity was positively correlated with the intensity of the experience reported by the participants. The stronger the experience, the higher the complexity!

Moreover, this study, led by Timmermann and published in 2019, also explored the different types of brainwaves (alpha, beta, theta, delta, gamma) and found that the increase in complexity was inversely correlated with the intensity of alpha brainwaves.[6] As we will see later on, these *alpha* waves seem to collapse during the psychedelic experience.

Although the role of alpha waves is complicated and remains a major enigma, these waves are most abundant during periods of mind wandering, and some studies suggest that they originate in the medial areas of the default network. It is also believed that they might exert a regulatory role over the spontaneous activity of more primitive areas.

As we will see throughout the book, the dominant theories regarding psychedelics' mechanism of action suggest that the observed changes in the visual cortex's behavior could be the indirect result of the effects that these molecules exert on both higher-order associative areas and over thalamic regulation.[7] For example, it has been suggested that the increased complexity of signals in the visual cortex could be a consequence of alpha-wave collapse. However, some people, such as my friend Marco Aqil, in a 2023 paper published with Leor Roseman, argue that we should not rule out the fact that the visual effects, at least those of a simpler nature, may also be in part the result of the direct stimulation of these molecules over the visual cortex. We will explore the basis for this theory in the next chapter.

Synesthesia

Another sensory phenomenon that is quite common during the psychedelic experience is the merging of different senses into one. Some people experience this phenomenon, called synesthesia, spontaneously, since it is hereditary and relates to how the brain develops in the first years of life. When the brain is formed, cortical neurons are connected in a rather homogeneous way. Then, by eliminating those synapses that are not useful and reinforcing those that are, the brain becomes "sculpted" by the first experiences in life. In synesthetes, it appears that some brain areas that normally become separated through day-to-day experience, remain neuroanatomically connected. Some researchers, such

---

6. See chapter 1 discussion of EEG and MEG.
7. See chapter 1 section on the regulation of thalamic activity.

as Vilayanur S. Ramachandran from the University of California, San Diego, suggest that this is possibly due to some genetic factor involved in neuroplastic processes.[8] The result is that a person who experiences synesthesia between numbers and colors, for example, will always process those two stimuli together. Since they both share the same brain signal, they become inseparable within the experience.

During the psychedelic experience, nonsynesthetes also have such experiences. For example, music is often accompanied by visuals, although many other combinations are possible: colors that are heard, tastes or sensations that are seen, words that are felt, and so on.

We do not know what causes the phenomenon of psychedelic synesthesia. To the best of my knowledge, there are no studies directly exploring it; but, as we shall see in the next chapter, it could be the result of changes in the regulatory mechanisms of the thalamus. If the usual segregation of sensory information within this structure is lost, it will send mixed signals to the sensory cortices. This is pure speculation. It could, for example, also be due to direct effects occurring at the sensory cortices.

Cognitive Effects

Visual effects are only a small fragment of the phenomenological changes promoted by psychedelics. Equally surprising are the effects occurring at the cognitive level. During the psychedelic experience, both the meaning of things (semantic effects) and the way in which information is manipulated (executive effects) change. Ultimately, the way in which thoughts unfold is abruptly transformed. This is extremely conspicuous and can lead to confusion.

Semantic Effects: Insight and Ego-Dissolution

Human beings are the only "linguistic animals" on the planet. Without a doubt, language is an integral part of our nature.

The science focused on studying how the brain generates and organizes meaning is called semantics. To study such processes, this discipline

---

8. Processes through which brain connections are sculpted. See chapter 1 (figure 4) on neuroplasticity.

has designed complex laboratory tasks that, by using words that have varying degrees of association between them, measure performance under different experimental conditions. For example, imagine a task in which one has to name a word displayed on the screen (i.e., target word) and that word is preceded by a different word (i.e., preceding word or distractor word). What effect does the degree of association between the target word and the preceding word have on the time it takes the participant to retrieve the target word from memory and respond to the task? This discipline has shown that the retrieval of the target word is facilitated when the preceding word is highly associated with the target word, which seems to indicate that the preceding concept activates the area of the semantic network where the target word is located. We could also say that the preceding word positions the system in a state proximal to the "final" state (corresponding to the target word). Thus, given that the preceding word "prepares" the area of the semantic map where the target word is located, the transition from the preceding state to the target state does not take much energy or much time. In short, it seems that the concepts within the semantic system form a complex and abstract network organized according to the degree of association between them, and that the activation of a representation spreads throughout the network, activating other representations following their degree of association.

When semantic tasks have been performed in the psychedelic state, results show significant differences in task performance. This suggests that the semantic network changes during this altered state of consciousness. For example, in a collaboration between the University of Kaiserslautern and Imperial College London, a study led by Neiloufar Family found that more mistakes were made during the altered states when participants were presented with highly associated words. Another study by Natasha Mason from Maastricht University reveals an increased ability to give alternative uses to everyday objects one week after the psychedelic session. This suggests that the psychedelic experience promotes unusual associations between semantically distant concepts. Although few studies have thus far been conducted, the results suggest that psychedelics disrupt the semantic network in a way in which the brain's associative capacity is widened.

Logically, the disruption of the semantic network impacts the nature of the representations, as well as their perception. During the psychedelic experience, meanings that we deal with daily are deconstructed and lose their familiarity. And beliefs that we previously took for granted are suddenly questioned, promoting the emergence of profound realizations, which by allowing us to think "outside the box" through which we usually process information, transform our way of understanding things.

It is not uncommon for people to express how psychedelics facilitated the detection and release of false premises, allowing them to transform, and thereby improve, a model or idea that they had strongly held before the experience. For example, Steve Jobs openly admitted that it was LSD that sparked his creativity and led to the creation of Apple. Or Francis Crick, who won a Nobel prize for identifying the structure of the DNA double helix, also recounted how LSD contributed to this three-dimensional view of DNA. And did you know that the dreaded PCR, yes, the technique applied when they stick that damn stick up our noses to detect COVID-19, is also the fruit of psychedelic inspirations? Its inventor, Kary Mullis, believes he would not have been able to invent such a thing had he not been using these substances.

However, although there are plenty of anecdotal reports, attempts at formally studying the supposed phenomenon of increased creativity, both during and after the psychedelic experience, have failed to point to any clear direction. Some studies have found an increase in certain creativity measures, whereas others have found a decrease, and multiple studies have found nothing.

Problems that are commonly encountered when attempting a scientific study of psychology might explain this. On the one hand, creativity is a very broad concept, and it does not have a unique and delimited definition: what specific aspect of creativity do we want to measure? What cognitive task will we use to measure such aspects? Often, the cognitive tasks designed are not capable of accurately detecting the concept being studied, or they only measure some aspects of the phenomenon and not others, limiting what we desire to know. Moreover, performance is logically affected by the participants' motivation toward the creative task.

To control for this last problem, a study described by James Fadiman in his book *The Psychedelic Explorer's Guide* was carried out in the 1960s on participants who were highly motivated to solve a specific problem related to their profession. Among them, there were engineers, mathematicians, physicists, and designers. Unfortunately, the U.S. Drug Enforcement Agency halted all human research using these substances and this study could not be completed. It only reached the phase of a pilot study and, for this and other reasons described by Matthew Baggott in *Psychedelics and Creativity: A Review of the Qualitative Literature*, the results are not entirely reliable. However, although the methodology and the way in which the study was reported were not ideal, we can use some of the participants' statements regarding how the deconstructive capacity of psychedelics allowed them to develop their creativity. Thus, for example, one participant said the following:

> I returned to the original problem. . . . I tried, I think consciously, to think of the problem in its totality, rather than through the devices I had used before.

And another said:

> I dismissed the original idea entirely and started to approach the graphic problem in a radically different way. That was when things started to happen. All kinds of different possibilities came to mind. . . .

This deconstruction and revision of beliefs has no limits, reaching the most fundamental of all beliefs: the belief about oneself.

Imagine that. To stop perceiving the conscious experience through the usual lenses of your identity. Yes, there is still an experience, but you are not there. The "I" as the observing subject of the experience remains, but the "me" as the perceived object, that semantic self that contains each one of your qualities (e.g., punctual, tidy, smoker, depressive, and the like), the one that dominates the mental narrative and tells you how to react and who to be, that "me," becomes more and more flexible until it disappears and stops making sense.

And, if you think about it, that semantic self, that identity, is highly linked to the judgmental and motivational functions of the limbic system.

The judgmental part manifests itself as we continually judge situations ("James is so rude!"). Such judgments are dictated by that which our identity finds meaningful and determined by how we should feel and act according to the belief of who we are ("We were supposed to meet at four o'clock. I can't stand people being late. I'm so angry! Next time it will be me who keeps him waiting. He will learn a lesson that way!").

On the other hand, the motivational part of our identity manifests itself through the goals we set for ourselves, through our desires, those which specifically activate our reward system and go beyond food, drink, sex, and company. Some of us want to travel, some of us want to write, some of us want to dance, some of us want to care for others. Each of us is motivated by different things, and our goals are largely shaped by the idea we have constructed of ourselves.

Although this idea of ourselves is, in part, possibly determined by the temperament with which we come into the world and by our childhood experiences, our identity is, for the most part, a reflection of the interpretations we have made of our experiences and by the stories we tell ourselves. Although our identity may gradually change, it is undoubtedly endowed with a certain stability. Yes, we have access to a wide repertoire of behaviors, depending on each specific situation and the state of mind in which we find ourselves at a certain moment. However, it is undeniable that our behavior is trapped within certain limits imposed by our identity. Or so we believe and feel until psychedelics dissolve it, and, by breaking down the barriers that separate the self from the world, connect us to "the whole."

It is not difficult to understand why the psychedelic experience may be therapeutic for people whose identities are trapped inside harmful thought patterns and behaviors. This experience can momentarily free them from the habitual chains of their mind and associated behaviors. By allowing them to observe themselves from a distance, a new perspective can be gained regarding both their flaws and virtues. This allows maladaptive beliefs about oneself, others, and the world to be transformed. In fact, the first study on treatment-resistant depression conducted by Imperial College London found that the levels of insight[9] (a phenomenon which is common during the mystical experience) achieved during the psychedelic session, correlated positively with the improvement in depressive symptoms five weeks after the experience. And look at how one of the smokers in a qualitative study led by Tehseen Noorani described how his identity was transformed and how such transformation enabled him to quit smoking:

> It felt like I'd died as a smoker and was resurrected as a nonsmoker. Because it's my perception of myself, and that's how I felt. So, I jumped up and I said "I'm not a smoker anymore, it's all done."

What areas of the brain do you think might be affected under the psychedelic experience, given these effects on one's identity and other more general meanings? Do you remember the default mode network described in chapter 1, that functional network removed from the perceptual world and involved in the higher-order representations regarding the inner world of concepts, beliefs, and identity? It turns out that during the psychedelic experience the different areas of the brain that were previously highly synchronized, giving this network its functional structure, become desynchronized and no longer share a common signal. The default mode network seems to dissolve. However, as we shall see, it seems that the dissolution of the ego goes beyond what happens in the default network.

The Default Mode Network and the Medial Temporal Lobe

Let's look at some of the neuroimaging results in more detail. Given its high activation during tasks that require us to reflect on ourselves, a study by Imperial College London led by Robin Carhart-Harris researched psilocybin-related connectivity changes in the medial prefrontal node of the default mode network in healthy adults.

---

9. During moments of insight there is a learning that comes through a profound revelation. It is important to mention that, although this often contains valuable and truthful information, there can also be moments of insight in which something is learned that, although appearing to be true, is objectively false.

On the top of color plate 16,[10] you can see the connectivity map of the default mode network's mediofrontal node under placebo, which clearly reveals the whole of the default mode network. When researchers compared the medial prefrontal cortex's connectivity map under placebo to the one obtained under psilocybin, they found that the mediofrontal node of the network became significantly disconnected from the posterior node located at the back of the cingulate cortex, the default mode network's main highway. In other words, the map below (psilocybin > placebo) shows a subtraction between the connectivity map obtained with the placebo and the connectivity map obtained with psilocybin, revealing the differences between the two connectivity maps.

The degree of disconnection between these areas did not correlate with the intensity of ego dissolution experienced under psilocybin

Placebo

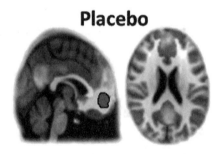

Psilocybin > Placebo

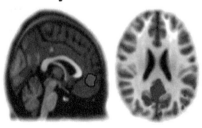

Figure 38. Changes in medial prefrontal cortex connectivity. The *top* row shows the connectivity map during the placebo. The *bottom* row shows a subtraction of the map obtained with placebo and the map obtained with psilocybin (psilocybin > placebo), showing the specific changes in the connectivity map of this prefrontal area due to psychedelics. Areas with which the medial prefrontal cortex loses connectivity are shown. Image taken from Carhart-Harris et al., published in *Frontiers in Human Neuroscience* in 2014. (See also color plate 16.)

---

10. Image modified from the following article: Carhart-Harris RL, Leech R, Hellyer PJ, Shanahan M, Feilding A, Tagliazucchi E, Chialvo DR, Nutt D. 2014. The entropic brain: a theory of conscious states informed by neuroimaging research with psychedelic drugs. Frontiers in Human Neuroscience 8:20.

reported by participants. However, Franz. X Vollenweider's team at Zurich University also found reduced functional connectivity between the frontal and posterior areas of the default mode network in a study in 2019 carried out in the context of a meditation retreat where some participants, who were all meditators, were given psilocybin. In this study, which was led by Lukasz Smigielski, no fMRI was taken during the altered state, but the day after the psychedelic experience, the connectivity between the frontal and posterior areas of the default mode network during an open-focus meditation task was weaker in those meditators who had taken psilocybin than in those who hadn't. Unlike focused attention meditation, in which one must sustain attention on a single object, open-focus meditation trains attention to move from one object to another without being trapped by any of them, something that should be highly beneficial for depressed patients who, as we will see, live trapped inside their minds and have a highly inflexible attentional focus. Moreover, Smigielski's team found that the observed magnitude between these areas' connectivity during open-focus meditation was correlated with the intensity of ego-dissolution experienced during the altered state of consciousness the previous day. Finally, the persistence of positive effects was measured four months later, and they found that these positive effects correlated with the intensity of ego dissolution achieved during the psychedelic trip.

This study was conducted on meditators instead of on depressed people, and the results were obtained during an open-focus meditation task. It's therefore a long shot, but could these results be, in some way, suggesting that psychedelic ego dissolution promotes changes in the default mode network that relate to an open-focused state of awareness? This could be tremendously beneficial for depressed patients. Of course, in order to explore this potential mechanism of action, we will need to develop experiments focused specifically on researching how the psychedelic experience impacts the attentional dynamics of depressed people. We will focus on depression in more detail when we study the emotional component of the psychedelic experience. For now, let's continue studying the possible neural correlates of psychedelic ego dissolution.

This time using MEG instead of fMRI, a 2013 study by Suresh D. Muthukumaraswamy from Carhart-Harris's team (2013) found that the ego dissolution reported by the participants was correlated with the reduction in the alpha waves picked up from the electrodes situated around the posterior node of the default mode network. Since brain waves emerge from the synchronization between local groups of neurons, these results suggest that the desynchronization between signals from this area is playing an important role in the ego-dissolution phenomenon.

We have already commented that alpha waves are possibly exerting a regulatory role over the spontaneous activity of the cortex and that their appearance has been associated with the medial areas of the default network.

Recall, for example, how in Timmermann's 2019 DMT study, the collapse of these alpha waves was inversely related to the increased complexity in the visual cortex's signals. Furthermore, as far as this section is concerned, the appearance of alpha waves has been associated with the controlled access of mnemonic information from the medial temporal lobe during ordinary states of consciousness (recall figure 19 in chapter 1 where you can see the location of these areas). This indicates that they may be regulating the spontaneous activity of hippocampal areas associated with delta and theta waves characteristic of REM sleep and of memory retrieval. With this in mind, it is interesting to note that under the effects of DMT, Timmermann not only finds that the collapse of alpha waves is inversely related to the increased complexity of signals from the visual cortex, but that the greater the collapse in alpha, the greater the emergence of medial temporal lobe-related delta/theta waves, suggesting that, medial temporal lobe activity is unleashed as midline alpha waves collapse.

Experiments in the 1960s had already linked the mystical experience to the activity of the medial temporal lobe. At that time, it was also discovered, that surgical ablations of this brain region suppressed psychedelic effects, as well as the fact that epileptic seizures originating in this brain area could generate the spontaneous emergence of mystical experiences. With this in mind, in addition to studying the behavior of the medial prefrontal cortex seen in figure 38, the Imperial College group also studied the behavior of the parahippocampal cortex during the psychedelic experience (you can find its location in figure 19, from

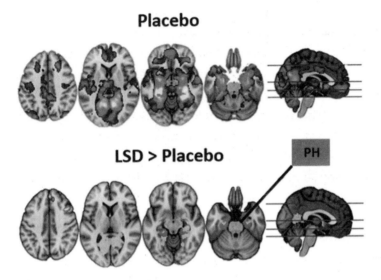

Figure 39. Changes in the connectivity map of the parahippocampal cortex (PH). The *top* row shows the connectivity map during the placebo. The *bottom* row shows a subtraction of the map obtained with the placebo and the map obtained with psilocybin, showing the specific changes in the connectivity of this limbic area due to LSD. Areas with which it loses connectivity are shown. Image obtained from Carhart-Harris et al., 2016, and published in *Proceedings of the National Academy of Sciences USA*. (See also color plate 17.)

chapter 1). The phylogenetically ancient structures of the medial temporal lobe are highly involved in the encoding and recollection of memories, and although Yeo's parcellation (presented in figure 28 in chapter 1) places them within the limbic network rather than within the default mode network, both networks work hand in hand and have a strong neuroanatomical connection. For example, as we saw when studying the limbic system, the limbic relay nucleus of the thalamus receives information from the hippocampus and projects to the orbitofrontal cortex and the posterior cingulate cortex,[11] the first area belonging, according to Yeo's parcellation, to the limbic network and the second, to the default network. In other words, although in Yeo's parcellation the default

---

11. You can see the diagram of this circuit in figure 20 and the location of these zones in figures 18, 19, and 30, all in chapter 1.

network and the limbic network form different networks, both are closely related through the limbic relay nucleus of the thalamus.

What did the researchers find when they studied the connectivity of the parahippocampal cortex during the psychedelic experience? In color plate 17[12] you can see the results. During the psychedelic experience, the parahippocampal cortex stops working so closely with the posterior cingulate cortex of the default network. It is, therefore, likely that the loss of connectivity between this medial temporal lobe area and the posteromedial areas of the default network, found in this study, is associated with Timmermann's 2019 findings relating the collapse of midline alpha waves to the emergence of theta/delta waves related to the medial temporal lobes.

The result in color plate 17 is particularly interesting, given that the decrease in connectivity between these areas was correlated with the level of ego dissolution reported by participants, similar to that which occurred with the reduction of alpha waves found in the posterior cingulate cortex using MEG. Is it possible that some changes in ego perception are due to primitive areas highly involved in episodic memory (located in the medial temporal lobe), ceasing to send information to the default network? This would prevent episodic information from reaching the frontal parts of this network (i.e., the medial prefrontal cortex) where the abstraction we have generated of ourselves, which we use to make decisions, resides.

This might be one of the mechanisms through which the ego dissolves, but it is worth mentioning that other studies show that the change in medial temporal lobe behavior does not seem to be limited to the cingulate cortex and the parahippocampal area (in figure 19 from chapter 1 you can see how the latter only represents a portion of the medial temporal lobe). Note that the results in color plate 17 were obtained by specifically studying the connectivity of one area (the parahippocampal area), which was selected a priori because of its relation to the mystical

---

12. Image modified from the following article: Carhart-Harris RL, Muthukumaraswamy S, Roseman L, Kaelen M, Droog W, Murphy K, Nutt DJ. 2016. Neural correlates of the LSD experience revealed by multimodal neuroimaging. Proceedings of the National Academy of Sciences USA 113(17):4853–4858.

experience described in the literature. However, by simultaneously study-ing changes in global connectivity (i.e., not just in one specific area) a 2015 study led by Alexander Lebedev from Karolinska Institutet and Stockholm University, Sweden found a more global effect that was not limited to the disconnection between the parahippocampal area and the posterior cingulate cortex. Rather, it appears that the entire medial tem-poral lobe (i.e., not just the hippocampal region) loses connectivity with broad regions of the associative cortex (i.e., not just with the posterior cin-gulate cortex). Beyond this, this study by Lebedev again found that the degree to which the medial temporal lobe loses connectivity with higher-order areas correlated strongly with the perceived level of ego dissolution. Something interesting is certainly happening during ego dissolution in this limbic and phylogenetically ancient area[13] involved in the encoding and retrieval of information!

The Insula

Dear reader, don't believe that the so-called ego dissolution can be understood so easily. It seems that it does not simply result from the disconnection between the medial temporal lobe and associative regions, nor by the disintegration of the default network. It would be much easier to write this book if that were the case! But I am afraid it is not. For example, some studies suggest that conventional antidepres-sants also produce connectivity changes within the default network, whereas we know that they do not produce the characteristic ego dis-solution obtained from high doses of psychedelics. Other mechanisms must be at play. And, in fact, the 2015 study by Lebedev mentioned above made an interesting finding that strongly implicated other areas outside the default network in ego dissolution.

Do you remember the insula?[14] Let's review its functions in more detail. This region is heavily involved in both monitoring the visceral state of the body and in the conscious processing of breathing, playing a

---

13. Phylogenetics is the study of the evolution of species and the relationship between them. Phylogenetically ancient areas are primitive areas, in this case the medial temporal lobe.

14. For more information on the insula, please refer to chapter 1.

key role in interoception. It also plays a fundamental role in promoting the feelings of agency[15] that lie behind the actions we take, as we saw in the introduction to the limbic system in chapter 1. When studying the functional networks described by Yeo (figure 28), Ledebev found that ego-dissolution's intensity was strongly correlated with the disintegration of the functional network containing this brain region (i.e., the salience network, described as the ventral attentional network in figure 28). Similarly, a collaborative study in 2016 by Enzo Tagliazucchi and Leor Roseman studying changes in global brain connectivity found that the disruption of the insula connectivity was also strongly related to the intensity of ego dissolution.

Although in Yeo's parcellation the insula doesn't belong to the somatic-sensory-motor network, we already know that, depending on the techniques and parameters used, different parcellations can be obtained, and how these are only approximations to the brain's intrinsic functional architecture. It turns out that a different method of parcellation was carried out in one of the analyses in Lebedev's study, obtaining a total of five networks. And, in this parcellation, the insula belonged to the same functional community as the somatic-sensory-motor cortex. It is not surprising that these two brain areas work so closely together when considering the insula's role in the feeling of agency and processing of bodily information. Let us then consider why the behavior of this area might be related to ego dissolution.

Could it, perhaps, be that the disintegration of the insular network contributes to modifying the more primitive and minimalist, prelanguage, body-related aspects of ego dissolution, whereas the effects observed in the default network are doing so by dissolving the more narrative and semantic aspects of the self? This interesting theory proposed by Lebedev will have to be investigated in more detail in future studies.

The above interpretation regarding the insula's implication in ego dissolution is centered around its bodily related functions, something we will return to when studying the corporal effects of these sub-

15. The sense of agency refers to the feeling that we are the authors (i.e., agents) behind the actions we take. For more information see section on the insula in chapter 1.

stances. But, given that this is a multifaceted structure, we could also relate the insula to the semantic effects promoted by psychedelics, and more specifically, to the phenomenon of insight. Let me explain why.

The insula is an extremely complex structure. As we discussed in chapter 1, in addition to its bodily functions, it is also involved in detecting personal relevant information, something it does through its close relationship with the ventromedial prefrontal cortex of the default network (limbic function), and with the anterior cingulate cortex of the ventral attentional network (cognitive function) (figure 24). But how does the assignment of relevance to a particular piece of information relate to having an insight?

We have already mentioned how these moments consist of profound realizations that are possibly facilitated by the relaxation of beliefs, but, what is it that exactly happens during these realizations? How does their inherent learning occur?

During an insight, learning does not necessarily occur by introducing new information into the system. Rather, what happens is that information that already exists within the system is restructured. More specifically, John Vervaeke (a passionate psychologist who has specialized in studying wisdom through a philosophical and cognitive approach, and creator of an exquisite YouTube channel[16] that I encourage anyone interested in human behavior and suffering to visit) believes that during moments of insight, there is a shift in the levels of relevance assigned to information within the system. According to Vervaeke, learning takes place when the system becomes reorganized according to shifts in the relevance maps.

We can find an example of this in episode 145 of Lex Friedman's podcast.[17] Here, Matthew Johnson, the lead researcher in the psilocybin for nicotine addiction clinical trial conducted at Johns Hopkins University,

---

16. You can easily find the channel by searching for John Vervaeke on YouTube. Within this channel there are several different series, including fantastic meditation classes and a series on the evolution of thought going back to before the Greek philosophers and the crisis of meaning we are going through in the West (the series is called *Awakening from the Meaning Crisis*).

17. You can find this episode on YouTube.

talks about a participant who, through the psychedelic experience, gained absolute clarity regarding how giving up smoking was entirely in his hands, how it was fully dependent on him. This obvious information already existed before the experience, but it was so ingrained in him that it was being ignored. Through the psychedelic experience, it now became highly salient and gained tremendous relevance, causing the system's information to reorganize around it. What was the result of changing the smoker's relevance landscape? At last, a change in his behavior!

Vervaeke's interpretation of insight is very interesting in light of the results obtained on the insula. The relationship between this structure, ego dissolution, and the insight phenomenon will need to be studied in more detail in the future. What we do know is that the greater the ego dissolution, the greater the likelihood of having a moment of insight. Could the insula connectivity changes associated with ego dissolution relate to the restructuring of the system's relevance landscape?

The Angular Gyrus

The intensity of the ego-dissolution phenomenon has also been correlated with changes in the behavior of one more final area. Specifically, the study led by Tagliazucchi and Roseman, who did an analysis simultaneously looking at the whole brain (as opposed to selecting a particular area), found that ego dissolution correlated with connective disruption, not only of the insula but also of the angular gyrus.

Let's take a closer look at this area. The angular gyrus is located at an intersection between the temporal, occipital, and parietal lobes (see the circle in figure 40), and is involved in many higher cortical functions. In figure 40[18] you can also see how the default mode, ventral attentional (which contains the insula) and frontoparietal networks converge in this area. Could it be that ego dissolution is, therefore, related to the connective disruption between the parts of the brain that encode information about the state of the body (i.e., the ventral

18. Image modified from the following article: Yeo BT, Krienen FM, Sepulcre J, Sabuncu MR, Lashkari D, Hollinshead M, Roffman JL, Smoller JW, Zöllei L, Polimeni JR, et al. 2011. The organization of the human cerebral cortex estimated by intrinsic functional connectivity. Journal of Neurophysiology 106(3):1125–65.

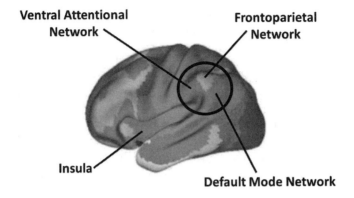

Ventral Attentional Network

Frontoparietal Network

Insula

Default Mode Network

Figure 40. Image of the Yeo networks showing the convergence between various high-order networks in the angular gyrus (marked by the circle). The location of the insular cortex is also shown. Image modified from a study led by Yeo and published in the *Journal of Neurophysiology* in 2011. (See also color plate 18.)

attentional network) and the parts of the brain that, using the episodic information of our life, encode the abstract idea we have generated of ourselves (i.e., the default network)?

Alternatively, recall that the angular gyrus is also highly involved in the spatial location of the body. Could ego dissolution also be linked to changes in the function of spatial location between the "I and the world?"

It will be difficult to disentangle the different components underlying this psychedelic phenomenon, but the genius of researchers is bound to surprise us.

Executive Effects

Let's turn now to the changes that these substances exert over the executive processes. During ordinary states of consciousness, the mind is constantly trying to solve problems by simulating possible scenarios. The processing and activation of information must be steered in a certain direction. That is, the activation of semantic information is usually directed by an end goal, whether conscious or unconscious, real or imagined. Such a goal will establish which information, among all the information available, needs to be integrated into a conscious experience and which needs to be suppressed. We refer to these as the "executive processes" and they are carried out by the attentional networks. A type of memory, working memory,[19] plays a key role, since it is here where the relevant information is maintained while it is being processed. Specifically, the frontoparietal network selects the relevant information for a given moment from the default network and other representational (i.e., perceptual) systems. Furthermore, such executive processes also help select and organize the actions required to fulfill the goal driving the individual.

We could say that during these ordinary states of consciousness we are in "doing" mode. But what happens when we launch into a psychedelic journey? Experiments using laboratory tasks designed to measure executive processes show that under the effects of these substances such abilities are seriously impaired. In this timeless state, our usual tendency of having to do something and solve problems becomes a big enigma for the individual. Its habitual meaning is lost. It is no longer understood.

One area heavily involved in such executive processes is the dorsolateral prefrontal cortex. Not surprisingly, when Carhart-Harris's team, from Imperial College, studied the connectivity of this area during a psychedelic experience, they observed significant changes in its behavior. At the top of figure 41,[20] you can see the connectivity map of this area (red spot in color plate 19) during ordinary states of consciousness. This map clearly corresponds to the frontoparietal executive network described by Yeo, a network highly involved in working memory. However, as the *bottom* row of figure 41 or color plate 19 shows, during the psychedelic experience, there is a clear disconnection between the frontal and parietal parts of this network. Although there are currently no studies that directly correlate this change in connectivity with performance on executive tasks, the disintegration of the frontoparietal network may lie behind the arduous work that maintaining and linearly manipulating information entails under psychedelic effects.

---

19. Working memory is equivalent to short-term memory.
20. Image modified from the following article: Carhart-Harris RL, Leech R, Hellyer PJ, Shanahan M, Feilding A, Tagliazucchi E, Chialvo DR, Nutt D. 2014. The entropic brain: a theory of conscious states informed by neuroimaging research with psychedelic drugs. Frontiers in Human Neuroscience 8:20.

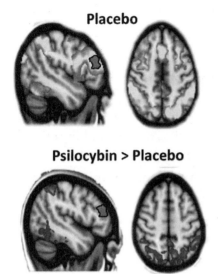

Placebo

Psilocybin > Placebo

Figure 41. Changes in the connectivity map of a central component of the frontoparietal executive network: the dorsolateral prefrontal cortex. Its usual connectivity map is shown at the *top*. At the *bottom*, its changes under psilocybin. Areas with reduced connectivity to the dorsolateral prefrontal cortex under psilocybin are also shown. Image obtained from Carhart-Harris et al., published in *Frontiers in Human Neuroscience* in 2014. (See also color plate 19.)

How might executive and semantic effects be related to ego dissolution? We don't have an answer, but I can think of two alternative possibilities. If, during ordinary states of consciousness, information is manipulated in a goal-directed manner, could these changes in executive processes be the result of the dissolution of the motivational parts of the self in charge of setting these goals? After all, as our identity dissolves, so does that which it desires. Although there is no evidence to sustain that said events are occurring in this direction, and although this explanation is, most likely, too simple and linear to be true, it is not a far-fetched hypothesis. However, the opposite might also be true: if executive processes in charge of manipulating information are affected by psychedelics, could this prevent the representation of oneself from being held in working memory, causing ego dissolution? Dear readers, this is what research is all about: an endless maze of circular questions, contradictions, much confusion, and, in the case of neuroimaging, an additional and problematic replication crisis. However, even though nothing is entirely clear to us, neuroimaging, coupled with these substances, undoubtedly helps us get a clearer picture of how the brain, this fascinating organ capable of generating conscious and idiosyncratic universes within each one of us, universes filled with stories, poetry, music, happiness, and suffering, works.

Mnemonic Effects

Let's turn now to another component of the psychedelic experience: its ability to transport us to particular places and times gone by. These vivid autobiographical memories, often accompanied by potent visuals, tend to gravitate around experiences that are highly emotional for the individual. And while they may evoke moments of great happiness, it is often the case that the person is transported back to some traumatic memory.

Bringing to light repressed traumatic memories can sometimes be tremendously beneficial, this being the basis of some schools of psychotherapy. But we must be cautious not to unconditionally accept the veracity of a supposed memory, as false memories are not uncommon. We know that memory is extremely fluid (much more so than it appears to be) and cannot always be relied upon, especially in the presence of suggestion, which increases under psychedelics. While, by helping the person modify their pathological beliefs and fill their life with new adaptive meanings, this suggestive capacity can be beneficial in psychotherapy, I must warn you, that in sectarian contexts, it can pose a great risk. Either way, regardless of the veracity of the memory and the dangers of suggestion, it will be important to use the integration sessions to try to decipher the underlying meaning that the perceived memory has for the individual (similar to that done with dreams).

When in the past the person has experienced a very stressful event in which their life was threatened, reliving such a traumatic experience in such a vivid way can promote a state of shock. In this case, the psychedelic experience could reinforce the past trauma rather than help in its resolution. It is for this reason, as Rosalind Watts reports on James Jesso's channel,[21] that therapists are considering the possibility of using lower, but still perceptible, doses of psychedelics in people with trauma-related depression.

How might psychedelics be promoting the re-experiencing of autobiographical memories? We know that mental imagery activates hip-

---

21. You can access this conversation on James Jesso's podcast "Adventures through the Mind."

pocampal brain areas and, as Nicholas W. Watkins has demonstrated, people with aphantasia,[22] who find it very difficult to evoke such imagery, have very poor autobiographical memories. This reinforces the notion that such mnemonic processes are closely linked to the visual system. Thus, given the pronounced autobiographical quality of this altered state of consciousness, it would make sense to observe changes in the behavior of parahippocampal and visual cortices. We already know that during the psychedelic experience, connectivity between the medial temporal lobe and associative cortices decreases and that this decrease correlates with ego dissolution. We also know that signals from the visual cortex spread throughout the brain promoting strong visuals. But how is the relationship between the medial temporal lobe and the visual cortex affected during the psychedelic experience? Some studies give us some interesting answers.

In one of these studies, once again led by Carhart-Harris and published in 2012, participants were asked to select several positive autobiographical memories in order to later recollect them inside a functional magnetic resonance imaging scanner. When researchers compared brain activity as the selected autobiographical memories were being recalled, they did not find an increased activity in the hippocampal areas under the effects of psilocybin. In both conditions (i.e., placebo and psilocybin) hippocampal activity was high, but this is not surprising, given that it was an autobiographical recall task, which, as we know, activates medial temporal lobe areas. However, they did find greater activation in visual and somatosensory areas during memory recall in those who were under the effects of psilocybin, as well as higher scores on visual vividness and intensity. It, therefore, seems that activation of primary cortices plays an important role when we recall an experience under the effects of a psychedelic and also points to the close relationship between such activation and the memory's vividness.

The other study that sheds some light on this question was published in 2016 and led by Mendel Kaelen, director and founder of Wavepaths, a

---

22. People with aphantasia have a reduced ability to visually represent images in their mind.

platform designed to travel inward by using the power of music. Given its ability to evoke emotions, music is being used extensively in psychedelic-assisted therapy, and we know that a synesthetic phenomenon between music and visuals often occurs. Based on this knowledge, this study explored medial temporal lobe connectivity while participants listened to music and found that, during the psychedelic experience, connectivity between the medial temporal lobe and the visual cortex increased. Moreover, the greater the increase in connectivity, the greater the visuals, particularly those of an autobiographical nature. Thanks to these studies we can now get a better picture of why autobiographical memories are experienced so vividly under psychedelics!

In short, it appears that during this altered state of consciousness, connectivity between the medial temporal lobes and the associative areas decreases, while connectivity to the primary areas increases.

Additionally, we have already seen how a study led by Chris Timmermann measuring brainwave changes under the effects of intravenous DMT found an increase in waves that are normally associated with the medial temporal lobe (delta/theta), and that this increase was correlated with both the peak of the experience and the collapse of alpha waves. Theta waves are associated with REM sleep, and, like the psychedelic experience, REM sleep is characterized by autobiographical overtones and detailed scenarios as well as being highly influenced by our unconscious. In fact, given that the psychedelic experience has a strong dreamlike quality, some have compared this state of consciousness to that of lucid dreaming. The appearance of theta waves makes perfect sense when considering this!

Emotional Effects

Psychedelics amplify our emotions as they lead us on an intense tour through the emotional content of our subconscious. This has nothing to do with the mechanism of action of conventional psychotropic drugs, which artificially dampen stress and mitigate the patients' inner struggle just about enough for them to be functional. Rather than facilitating the avoidance of difficult emotions, psychedelics, instead, put us face to face with them. As such, they can undoubtedly lead us to the darkest corners of our psyche, to those nooks and crannies buried by the ego's defense mechanisms. The psychedelic experience can make us feel what seems like humankind's collective sadness or painful and intense feelings of guilt, fear, or paranoia.

This, combined with the potential confusion that the deconstruction of meanings may produce, can be extremely stressful and lead to "bad trips," prolonged states of dissociation, or even psychotic breaks when done in chaotic and uncontrolled settings. However, clinical studies suggest that, by freeing us from the usual frames imposed by the fears of our ego, in controlled settings and under the supervision of experienced therapists, the emergence of difficult emotions can be navigated fruitfully, allowing us to work on such challenging contents in a novel way that can be particularly therapeutic.

Moreover, during the psychedelic experience, provided the environment and intention are appropriate, this emotional tour through the psyche is often accompanied by an, often forgotten or even unknown, feeling of self-compassion.

This self-compassion protects and supports us as we try, by facing the threatening task of confronting those parts of ourselves that burden us with guilt, shame, and dissatisfaction, to illuminate the darkness of our shadow. We are not yet able to determine the causality between the different effects of psychedelics. However, this self-compassion likely plays a central therapeutic role as, by discovering within ourselves this part that is capable of loving and caring for the damaged parts, these can, at last, begin to transform and heal.

See how beautifully one of the depressed patients in a qualitative study led by Rosalind Watts described the way in which such self-compassion presented itself during their experience:

I had an encounter with a being, with a strong feeling that that was myself, telling me it's alright, I don't need to be sorry for all the things I've done. I had an experience of tenderness towards myself. During that experience, there was a feeling of true compassion I had never felt before.

And these feelings of compassion go beyond oneself. Watts comments on how several of her patients described "love" as a powerful supernatural force. That powerful force that you feel within yourself that cares for others, reaches out to those who have hurt you, allowing you to forgive and release the resentment you carry within.

In short, these substances tend to address the root of our pain in a similar way to some psychotherapies, but by promoting self-compassion and so abruptly lowering the ego's defense mechanisms, they have an added capacity, that neither psychotherapy nor conventional psychotropic drugs have. In this state, the weakened ego struggles to maintain the frequent mollifying avoidance of emotions, that defense mechanism that so often ends up worsening the wounds we carry. Instead, the release of powerful emotional catharsis, a key to alleviating psychic discomfort, is enabled.

An online study led by Leor Roseman corroborates how the effects these substances have on emotional processes mediate their therapeutic potential. Nearly four hundred participants filled out questionnaires about the emotional content of the psychedelic trip experienced the day before. Researchers found that it was common for psychonauts to report having faced and released normally avoided and repressed emotions, resolved personal conflicts, and obtained a sense of relief. Particularly interesting is the fact that, in the seventy-five patients who two weeks before the session presented low levels of well-being, the degree to which they had experienced such emotional release was predictive of improved well-being two weeks after the psychedelic experience.

Similarly, while before the psychedelic session the depressed patients in Rosalind Watts' study reported feeling disconnected and trapped in their mind, after their trip they explained how "the mental fog" had cleared or how "the lights had come on," feeling clarity and a broad mental space, whereas before, they only felt the crushing sensation caused by "rumination." In short, people who previously felt a deep isolation and disconnection now felt part of the world, interacting more, not just with other people, as this patient comments:

> I was talking to strangers. I had these full long conversations with everybody I came into contact with.

But, also, with other stimuli from the environment, as the words of this other person show:

When I went outside, everything was very bright and colourful and it felt different. I noticed things I didn't notice usually, the leaves on the trees and the birds, small details.

And an awesome connection with every other human being, according to this other patient:

I would look at people on the street and think "how interesting we are." I felt connected to all of them.

But, in a more fundamental way, patients reported feeling more connected to themselves, to the person they were before the depression, and they also reported feeling a greater sense of worth and confidence, as well as a greater determination to become the person they wanted to be. They had reprogrammed their identity.

When, instead of depressed patients, Tehseen Noorani has qualitatively studied the experiences of the smokers who participated in the Johns Hopkins University study, it has been found that they also gained profound realizations that helped them quit smoking. Some, about how their true identity did not need to incorporate cigarettes and about how they were perfectly capable of quitting smoking. Others, about their true values regarding how they should prioritize health over the urge to smoke. And several reported how, in the face of immense universal interconnectedness, tobacco, once an integral part of their persona, now became insignificant. But, in addition, and in relation to this particular section of this chapter, of the twelve participants interviewed, three referred to tobacco as a friend, and two of them mentioned how smoking helped them connect with people, suggesting that addictive behaviors might emerge from feelings of disconnection, something that has also been supported by experiments with rats.

Between the 1960s and 1980s, a purely biological model of addiction based on the behavior of rats that had been isolated in tiny cages was developed. These rats were given the option of drinking water from two bottles, one of which contained heroin. Under these conditions, the rats developed addictive and compulsive behavior until they eventually overdosed and died.

At this time the biomedical approach prevailed, so the researchers of these studies did not consider the huge impact that the environmental conditions could be having on the rodent's behavior, concluding that the biological properties of substances such as heroin or cocaine must irremediably turn us into addicts. However, suspecting that the highly artificial environment in which these animals were kept might be affecting the results, in the late 1970s, Bruce K. Alexander's team set up a series of experiments at Simon Fraser University in British Columbia whose results ended up revolutionizing our understanding of addictive behavior.

In these studies, the researchers offered the rats the same drinking options as in previous studies but did not isolate them in small cages. Instead, they created a large recreational park, the "Rat Park," where the animals could entertain themselves with various environmental stimuli (empty cans to hide in, wood to chew on, platforms to climb, wheels to run on, and so on) and interact and copulate with other rats, finding, through these studies, that addictive behavior did not emerge within such an enriched environment. Yes, the rats occasionally chose to drink the heroin water but did so only recreationally. Not one single case of overdose was recorded. In this new environment, heroin did not seem to behave like the biological monster that had been portrayed in previous studies. What would happen, then, if isolated and addicted rats who should be biologically dependent on the substance were introduced into this new environment? Surprisingly, and contrary to the prognosis established by the theories on addiction at the time, the rats reversed their addictive behavior in the new environment. Incredible!

Although the Rat Park results had enormous implications and showed the huge experimental error that had been made by using isolated rats, the scientific community did not grant these results the immediate recognition that they deserved. In retrospect, it seems absurd that it took so long to recognize how silly it was to study the behavior of social animals in such an artificially confined environment. But I suppose this is just a reflection of those innate mechanisms that, to provide us with a certain stability, maintain us in the grip of our beliefs.

Fortunately, the Rat Park studies have finally succeeded in transforming the previous biomedical approach to addiction into a new biosocial one that includes, as the name suggests, social as well as biological factors. This has been a huge step forward and has even led to legislative changes in some countries. If isolation causes addictive behavior, what sense does it make to try to eliminate this problematic behavior by locking people up in cages? In 2000, Portugal, at the forefront of countries that have changed their drug policy, shifted from treating substance abuse as a criminal problem to treating it as a mental health one, decriminalizing drug use. Since then, money previously earmarked for criminal spending has been directed to psychological support programs for users and, according to an analysis by the New York Times, seventeen years after implementing these policies, the number of heroin users had fallen from 100,000 to 25,000 people. Clearly, the programs seem to be working, which begs the question of why other countries are not following suit.

The world is full of stimuli, and the brain has evolved to interact with them, process them, and release a certain, and optimal, amount of neurotransmitters. Isolated in cages, the rats had no access to pleasurable stimulation, heroin being the only environmental stimulus capable of (through its action on opioid receptors) generating a dopamine release that would activate the animal's reward system.[23] Pleasure seeking and pain avoidance are two of the most primitive mechanisms since life began on Earth, and being caged in such a poor and confined space meant that the animal was not able to go in search of different rewarding stimuli. It is logical then that in these conditions, the rats would become obsessed with the only stimulus capable of providing them with pleasure. Of course, due to the poor environment, once this obsessive drug

---

23. See the section on the neuroanatomy of the limbic system from chapter 1 regarding the striatum.

consumption is triggered, changes in the distribution of dopaminergic and opioid receptors in neuronal membranes are produced, which end up causing withdrawal symptoms in the absence of the pleasurable stimulus. And once the animal has reached this point, consumption no longer involves obtaining pleasure, but rather the elimination of pain, prompting it to compulsively seek the drug in order to calm its discomfort.

The psychological implications of human social behavior certainly make it much more complex than that of other social animals. But even so, and even, considering the transformations that phylogenetically older mechanisms and structures[24] undergo as they continue to evolve, our behavior undoubtedly shares some basis with that of other animals in our phylogenetic lineage. If you are a follower of Jordan Peterson, a clinical psychologist and former professor at the University of Toronto, famous for his role in the cultural war of ideas of the moment, you might be thinking about how the posture that lobsters adopt depending on their perceived hierarchical position is related to the serotonergic system, and how this might still be the case in humans, something Jordan Peterson describes in his lessons from lobsters.

Be that as it may, even on these common grounds, it is still difficult to translate the results of addictive behaviors in rodents to human behaviors, but we can nonetheless try. Let's do it.

Could addictive behavior in humans be a symptom of the loneliness felt by the individual? Could this sense of isolation be hindering the ability to interact with the world and derive satisfaction from it and the social relationships inherent to our society? Could obsessive behavior over that which artificially activates our reward system be the consequence of not deriving pleasure from any other sources? I don't know much about biosocial theories of addiction, but if this is the case, it would make sense to think that the connection promoted by psychedelics would be therapeutic in treating addictive behaviors.

We humans love to let the world know who we are, to be known. A desire much exploited by social networks such as Facebook. The need

24. Recall that phylogenetics refers to the branch of science that studies the evolutionary relationship between different species. Phylogenetically ancient structures therefore refer to primitive brain structures that, for example, we share with reptiles.

to socialize and be seen is anchored deep in our nature, and thus we naturally suffer and develop psychopathological behaviors when we feel lonely! Several studies have found that after a psychedelic experience, empathy and prosocial behavior increase in a lasting way. Through a good psychedelic experience, people not only discover many parts of themselves that accompany them at all times. They also discover a whole three-dimensional world to explore, a world full of beauty to actively participate in and share with other beings and other beings to interact with, to become part of the other and the other part of oneself, thus managing not only to transform oneself through others but also to *share oneself* with them. In short, after a good psychedelic experience, a person can finally stop feeling lonely and receive satisfaction from the world. That said, there are limits to what a good psychedelic experience can achieve. If the environment one returns to is toxic, the suffering will continue. However, the teachings gained from the psychedelic experience can arm us with tools with which to deal better in such an environment, and energy with which to fight to change it, or at least not make it worse.

What effects do neuroimaging studies observe when looking into the limbic system during and after the psychedelic experience? How might the observed changes be benefitting people with maladaptive behaviors?[25] Be warned that we will now engage in an intense speculative exercise, but given the preliminary stage of this line of research, we have no other choice. Besides, that's research! Let's see what the studies find.

Stimuli used in tasks designed to study emotional processes often consist in the presentation of people's faces showing different facial expressions or of negative or positive words to which the participant has to react, measuring reaction times, errors made, or in the case of neuroimaging, neural responses during the task.

When these tasks have been carried out on healthy people under the effects of psilocybin, the results suggest that, at least in the safe and

---

25. Maladaptive behaviors are behaviors that cause some kind of problem for the individual such as reckless, addictive, or impulsive behaviors.

controlled environments in which such studies are conducted, psilocybin may interfere with the processing of negatively charged stimuli.

For example, it has been observed that under the effects of psilocybin, the processing of faces with negative facial expressions such as sadness or fear is harder than the processing of faces with happy expressions. Similarly, when instead of faces, reaction times to different words were measured, it was found that, under the effects of psilocybin, faster responses were obtained to positive words than to negative ones, showing once again that in this state it is easier to process positive than negative information. These behavioral results have been corroborated by a study in 2011 using EEG in healthy people. This study, led by Michael Kometer from the Heffter Research Institute, measured an electrophysiological signal called the P300 wave, which we know appears during attentional processes. The results showed an overall reduction in the magnitude of P300 under the effects of psilocybin, something which was to be expected, given the disruptive effects these molecules have on such attentional processes. However, this reduction was greater for negative stimuli than for positive ones, supporting the theory that psilocybin decreases the ability to attend to negative stimuli to a greater extent than to positive ones, at least in healthy people in safe environments.

The results observed under the effects of psychedelics are very significant, given that previous studies on depressed patients during ordinary states of consciousness show that they have shorter reaction times and higher P300 to negative words than to positive words (i.e., greater ease in the processing of negative than positive information). Could the observed results perhaps suggest that this hindrance in the processing of negative information is freeing them from their negative bias, thus helping depressed patients to improve their emotional regulation? By freeing up mental attentional spaces normally occupied by negative information, this increased difficulty in processing negative stimuli could be reversing their usual bias. But there is also another alternative. Perhaps, rather than being a direct effect of psychedelics, the decrease in negative bias could be an indirect consequence of the positive feelings promoted by the novelty of the experience. Either way, it seems that, at least in safe and controlled settings, there is less processing of negative information.

If you recall the limbic system from chapter 1, you are probably wondering about the amygdala. We know that this structure is highly involved in affective tasks and that, in people with depression and anxiety, it shows hyperactivity to negative stimuli. How does this structure behave during the psychedelic experience? Several neuroimaging studies have focused on looking closely at this.

Using functional magnetic resonance, two studies on healthy participants have found that when fearful faces are presented under the effects of psychedelics there is a reduced reactivity in this structure. Furthermore, in one study in 2009 led by Erik M. Mueller from Boston University, this reduction was correlated with the subjective effects of the psychedelic experience, and in another study from the University of Zurich led by Rainer Kraehenmann, it correlated with the improvement of mood at the end of the session. The lower the hyperactivity, the higher the intensity of the experience and the better the mood, respectively.

Given these results and the well-established link between the amygdala and fear and stress responses, one would intuitively expect to find that, following the psychedelic experience, depressed patients would show less activity in this structure when viewing negatively charged stimuli, right? Get ready to experience a neuroscientist's bread and butter, because, while in a Johns Hopkins University study led by Frederick Barrett on healthy participants, this is indeed what was found one week after the psychedelic session, the same outcome was not true in another study of depressed patients carried out by Imperial College. This study, led by Roseman, compared the amygdala reactivity to facial expressions the day after and the day before the psychedelic session and found a greater overall reactivity (i.e., to both positive and negative stimuli) the day after. You might wonder: A greater reactivity of the amygdala the day after the psychedelic experience despite having fewer depressive symptoms? And a lower reactivity in healthy patients a week later? It should be borne in mind that these two studies involved different populations and that in one study activity was measured a week later and in the other the day after. But, in principle, Roseman's results are still contradictory. I am afraid that the behavior of complex systems is often counterintuitive and solutions are never linear. But don't despair, we can speculate on possible explanations for this result.

It is perhaps important to note that the increased amygdala reactivity found in the study on depressed patients was not only found in response to negative facial expressions (and incidentally, the increase in this reactivity correlated with the improvement of symptoms one week later), but that there was also an increased reactivity to positive expressions. Remember now that depressed people live in a constant state of "rumination,"[26] which, despite causing high levels of stress, traps them in a dimension dominated by a mental narrative that occupies the attentional space needed to pause and feel emotions. Could these results perhaps point to the ability of the psychedelic experience to reconnect depressed people with their emotions and thus improve emotion regulation? This is what the researchers suggest, although this will need to be tested in a larger sample. If so, this is a very different mechanism of action than that of conventional antidepressants, which do appear to reduce amygdala reactivity to affective stimuli in depressed patients.

But don't relax. It's not that simple. Another Imperial College London study led by Carhart-Harris investigating brain activity during rest (i.e., without performing any task) did find that the day after psychedelic intake, depressed patients showed lower baseline activity in the amygdala, a reduction that was also correlated with improvement in depressive symptoms.

Does this mean that symptom improvement correlates with both increased amygdala reactivity to negative stimuli and decreased baseline amygdala activity in resting states? Assuming we can trust these results, which we should take with caution, given the present replication crisis that neuroimaging is going through and the small number of participants in the study, this seems to be the case. If reliable, and if the

---

26. In this state the person has obsessive thoughts about their distress and its causes, often revolving around some past event.

increased amygdala reactivity to positive and negative stimuli is indeed reflecting better emotional regulation, could these results be pointing at how the psychedelic experience reduces negative bias through reducing basal activity in the amygdala during rest, while at the same time improving emotional regulation by allowing greater contact with emotions? Many more studies will be needed to unravel all these questions and get clearer answers, and they should be on their way!

Furthermore, we know that the limbic system goes beyond the amygdala. In chapter 1 we saw how, in order to evaluate environmental information and make a decision, the amygdala communicates closely with both the sensory cortex and the prefrontal cortex. This communication is bidirectional, since there are both bottom-up and top-down projections between these structures, with the amygdala, positioned at the center of this circuit (figure 42). That is, on the one hand, the amygdala receives information from the sensory cortex and sends information to the prefrontal cortex (bottom-up processing). On the other hand, the prefrontal cortex regulates amygdala activity by sending projections that activate inhibitory neurons in this structure, and similarly, the amygdala sends regulatory projections to the sensory cortex (top-down processing).

Given this bidirectional circuit between the sensory cortex, the amygdala, and the prefrontal cortex, an increase in the amygdala's activity could mean several things. On the one hand, it could be reflecting activation of regulatory projections to the sensory cortex; but on the other hand, it could also be reflecting activation of ascending projections to the prefrontal cortex. Additionally, it could also be the result of a lack of inhibition by the prefrontal cortex, or, alternatively, be due to an excess of threatening input from the sensory

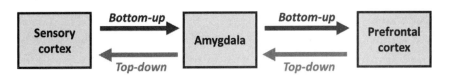

Figure 42. Schematic diagram of connections between the prefrontal cortex, the amygdala, and the sensory cortex.

cortex. Hence, we cannot only study the activity of this structure. It is essential to also study its connectivity and directionality.

Some studies in depressive patients suggest that conventional antidepressants such as escitalopram work, at least in part, by affecting the regulation that the prefrontal cortex exerts over the amygdala. But what about psychedelics? What part of this circuitry are they affecting? To answer this question, Kraehenmann's study in 2016 explored the connectivity between the visual cortex, the amygdala, and the lateral prefrontal cortex during the processing of "threatening" stimuli and applied a complex technique that allowed them to establish the directionality of this connectivity. Which aspect of this circuit was affected by psychedelics? The results seemed to show that, at least within the circuit formed by these three areas, during the processing of threatening information, psilocybin affected the top-down regulation that the amygdala exerted on the visual cortex.

What is the function of these top-down projections from the amygdala to the visual cortex? Imagine you are in the jungle, mesmerized by a beautiful flower, and suddenly a poisonous snake appears. This new visual information is threatening and extremely important so it will activate the amygdala. The top-down projections that the amygdala sends to the visual cortex allow this subcortical structure to quickly and unconsciously select which sensory information should rise to consciousness and which should not. In this case, this will push the information regarding the flower into the background and, in its place, detailed information about the snake will ascend to consciousness. The process of reorientation of attention and selection of information is of course much more complex than the unconscious regulation of the amygdala over the visual cortex. Conscious processes will involve attentional networks, namely, the frontoparietal control and the dorsal attentional network.

Ultimately, our emotional state is affected by incoming information, but it also determines the information we pay attention to, or instead ignore. People with anxiety or post-traumatic stress disorder are in a hypervigilant state, continually monitoring the environment for threats. Could psilocybin modulate people's negative biases, at least in part, by modifying the environmental information that the amygdala selects? According to the researchers, that may be what Kraehenmann's study suggests.

Despite the results from this study, we should not reject the possibility that psychedelics also work through increasing prefrontal cortex regulation over the amygdala. In Kraehenmann's study, these three areas (i.e., the amygdala, the visual cortex, and the lateral prefrontal cortex) were selected because they showed greater activity when viewing threatening stimuli than when viewing geometric shapes in an imaging analysis done before the psychedelic experience. However, the study that showed that conventional antidepressants did increase the regulation of the prefrontal cortex over the amygdala was focused on the orbitofrontal cortex and not the lateral one (see figure 17 from chapter 1 to locate these areas). As that figure shows, the prefrontal cortex encompasses many more areas than the lateral area studied by Kraehenmann's team and is highly involved in regulating the activity of subcortical structures. It would then be perfectly possible that, in a similar way to that of conventional antidepressants, psilocybin could be having an effect over the regulation that areas of the prefrontal cortex, different from the lateral one, exert over the amygdala, as Kraehenmann argues. Let us hope that this question is being studied already! For example, what would an analysis like the one used by Kraehenmann's team find when substituting the lateral cortex for the orbitofrontal one?

There are additional reasons to focus on the orbitofrontal cortex. For example, Frederick Barrett's team, from Johns Hopkins University, in 2020 found increased activity in this area during a task that presented emotionally conflicting stimuli to healthy participants one week after the psychedelic session. Perhaps this increased activity is reflecting this area's ability to control emotions and impulses in the face of the emotionally conflicting information presented in the task. The scientific community will have to repeat this experiment with depressed patients. If increased activation of the orbitofrontal cortex is once again found after the psychedelic experience, they'll have to explore whether it relates to top-down projections going to the amygdala as well as to symptom improvement.

Finally, two other studies in healthy patients have found that improved mood correlates with changes in connectivity between the amygdala and areas of the prefrontal cortex. For example, one study led by Oliver Grimm in 2018, from the team in Zurich, found that, under the effects of psilocybin, connectivity between these areas decreased when looking at happy faces, and that the greater the decoupling, the greater the positive mood. The other publication from 2020, led by Anya K. Bershad, studied brain connectivity under the effects of a microdose of LSD at rest and found that increased connectivity between the amygdala and the prefrontal cortex correlated with improved mood. Although microdoses are not detectable, some people follow specific protocols, such as those developed by James Fadiman or Paul Stamets, and take them regularly since they feel that these subtly improve their mood. Today, the few methodologically sound studies that have been carried out have found very few significant differences in people's emotional state after controlling for expectancy and placebo effects, and no promising differences during task performance. Bershad's study did, however, seem to find an effect on connectivity, suggesting that perhaps the effects of microdosing go beyond placebo and that, thus far, the other studies have failed to detect it.

Because Grimm's and Bershad's experiments did not study the directionality of such connectivity, we cannot draw any conclusions from their results. However, they do seem to support the notion that psychedelics promote the improvement of people's emotional state by modulating the connectivity between the amygdala and the prefrontal cortex during the psychedelic experience.

You may have noticed that so far, the above-mentioned studies exploring changes in the limbic system's connectivity were carried out in healthy patients. What happens then in depressed patients? Is there a change in amygdala connectivity after the psychedelic experience? The answer is that Carhart-Harris's study from 2017 on depressed patients, in which lower basal activity in the amygdala had been found the day after the psychedelic experience, found no changes in the amygdala's connectivity. Instead, the researchers found that improvement in depressive symptoms five weeks after the psychedelic session could be predicted by connectivity changes observed the day after the psychedelic session in two other areas highly involved in the limbic system: the hippocampus[27] (which appeared less connected to an area of the medial/lateral prefrontal cortex), and the ventromedial prefrontal cortex[28] (which appeared more connected to the angular gyrus[29]).The fact that these connectivity changes predicted the clinical improvement observed at five weeks makes these findings extremely interesting. What may they mean?

Let's start by speculating about the first outcome. We know that depressed people are trapped in a state of rumination characterized by thoughts that often revolve around some past event in which the person wishes they had acted differently. We also know that, during these thoughts, the person blames themselves for having acted the way they did. For example, someone may be obsessively trapped in the following thought: "why did I do that, I wish I had behaved differently! I'm pathetic." Thus, on the one hand, rumination requires the memory in question to be recalled, something we know involves the hippocampus and surrounding areas of the medial temporal lobe. And, on the other hand, it requires that a judgment be made about how the person acted in that episode, which we know requires the activation of the prefrontal areas within the default mode network, involved in determining how we should act according to the idea we have constructed of ourselves. Or in the case of rumination, how we should have acted. For this judgment to occur, it is, therefore, necessary for the hippocampus to send episodic information to the medial prefrontal cortex. Could it then be that the reduced communication between the hippocampus and the prefrontal cortex is reflecting the less repetitive evaluation of past episodes? Could it even be reflecting less obsession over the reprocessing of memories and instead more attention to information coming from the senses, and thus, to the present moment? It's a possibility!

What might the other result be indicating, which suggests that increased connectivity between the ventromedial prefrontal cortex and the angular gyrus after the psychedelic experience is beneficial for the

---

27. You can see the location of the hippocampus in figures 18 and 19 from chapter 1.

28. You can see the location of the ventromedial prefrontal cortex in figure 17 from chapter 1.

29. You can see the location of the angular gyrus in figure 40 from this chapter.

individual? The researchers decided to study connectivity changes in the ventromedial prefrontal cortex because of its high involvement in tasks involving the activation of one's identity.[30] Moreover, we have already discussed how this area, along with the orbitofrontal cortex and other areas of the prefrontal cortex, plays not only an important role in regulating emotions and impulses but that it also works closely with the insula, which is involved in assigning personal relevance to information (figure 24). Furthermore, we have discussed how relevance maps, through which we process information, determine what we pay attention to and the actions that we should take. Recall the participant who quit smoking after the revelation that quitting smoking was entirely in his hands (information that was already contained in the system but was not being made relevant before the trip). Could it, therefore, be that the ventromedial prefrontal cortex's connectivity is reflecting the changes that the relevance map goes through during moments of insight? Through the ventromedial prefrontal cortex's regulation of nucleus accumbens (impulses) and amygdala (emotions), the change in its relevance maps should modify the way a person behaves and deals with their emotions, which is critical in combating depression and addiction. But a question remains. Why is it that the connectivity increase occurs precisely between the ventromedial prefrontal cortex and the angular gyrus? I guess by this point in the book you can imagine that I don't have a clear answer for you, but a few ideas do come to mind.

Let's see, what do we know about the angular gyrus? We know that it is an area of convergence between the insular (i.e., ventral attentional), the default mode, and the frontoparietal networks (see figure 40 presented earlier in this chapter). This suggests that this area plays a fundamental role in coordinating activity between these high-order networks and thus directing attention, which has very little flexibility in obsessive, depressed, anxious, and addicted individuals. We also know that when, in healthy participants, connectivity changes of the whole brain were studied simultaneously, the greater the ego dissolution, the greater

---

30. Identity is understood as the representation that one has generated of oneself through which one decides how to act in different situations.

the connective disruption in this area of high-order network convergence. To the best of my knowledge, there is no study in a depressed population using the analysis that produced these results, but, if such connective disruption also occurs in depressed patients (which is likely), could it be allowing the pathological coordination between these three networks to be restructured as the ego is loosened?

Perhaps the increased connectivity between the ventromedial prefrontal cortex and the angular gyrus is reflecting the change in the way the new salience map, drawn in the ventromedial cortex, is modifying the person's attentional preferences. Let's go further. Given the important role that the angular gyrus plays in the spatial location of the self, the increased connectivity between these areas might even be reflecting the relevance that the outside world gains as the person begins to engage more with the environment after finally breaking free from their mind's prison. The great enigma surrounding how the brain works opens up an infinite number of questions and possibilities. Surely none of our possible explanations is the ultimate explanation, but it is nonetheless fascinating to try to decipher the mechanisms that give rise to the tremendous richness within human consciousness, something that, with the help of psychedelics, becomes an easier (relatively!) and more engaging task.

We cannot end this section without mentioning one last study. The tasks mentioned so far presented faces and emotionally charged words. While it is true that these stimuli manage to activate our limbic system through unconscious processes, they do not capture one of the things we humans fear most: the fear and pain associated with social exclusion, which is so accentuated in both depression and addictions. To study the mechanisms underlying such pain, psychologists have developed a computer task, the "Cyberball," in which the participant believes he or she is part of a team in which a ball is passed around. As the task unfolds, the researchers modify the degree to which the team includes or excludes the participant.

Using this task to explore which areas are activated when we feel excluded, it has been found that the anterior cingulate cortex is highly involved in these conditions. Recall that this area works closely with the insula, giving rise to the ventral attentional network, and that, as we saw in chapter 1, both are highly involved in the processing of psychic pain. How are the feelings of social exclusion and the activity of the anterior cingulate cortex affected when this task is performed under the effect of psychedelic molecules?

Using the Cyberball task in healthy patients, a study led by Katrin Preller from Zurich's team has shown that those participants taking psilocybin felt less excluded during the task than those taking the placebo. In addition, it was also found that when participants were being excluded, the anterior cingulate cortex was less activated under the effects of psilocybin. Finally, the activity of this area was correlated with the feeling of unity experienced during the psychedelic trip: the greater the feeling of unity, the lower the activation in this area, suggesting that the feelings of connection experienced in this state seem to be able to reverse the feelings of isolation and social exclusion that are so pronounced in some psychopathologies. This fantastic experiment by Zurich's team should be repeated in depressed and addicted patients!

Having reviewed the emotional effects and studies that have focused on exploring changes in the processing of affective information, you will appreciate that we still do not fully understand how psychedelics help people improve their emotional regulation. However, it does appear that these substances may make it easier to cope with difficult emotions and improve feelings of well-being. Socially they may also reduce feelings of isolation and social exclusion by promoting a sense of universal connectedness.

Although we are far from being able to set any theory in stone, the results reviewed in this section might suggest that the ease of coping with difficult emotions is linked to the fact that, during the psychedelic experience, the amygdala does not seem to react as strongly to material that is normally processed as threatening. However, it is important to emphasize here that anecdotes of psychedelic trips flooded with profound feelings of terror do abound. It is therefore unlikely that the reduction in amygdala reactivity is a direct pharmacological effect of psychedelics. Instead, it is more likely an indirect effect promoted by the subjective experience.

We know that the environment in which these molecules are consumed plays an essential role in determining the quality of the experience, and given the existence of psychedelic horror stories, it is likely to also affect the activity of the amygdala. Additionally, it is important to consider that the stimuli used in the tasks are far removed from real-life situations. Although such stimuli can activate unconscious mechanisms associated with fear, the faces and words in the tasks are not stimuli that one cognitively perceives as threatening. If, as the ego weakens, one does not feel safe enough to relax one's defensive barriers and present oneself "naked" to the world in the environment with which one is merging, a fear of a much more complex nature than that triggered by laboratory tasks will almost certainly appear. Whereas the fear elicited by laboratory tasks is based on unconscious and primitive processes, the fear elicited by more realistic situations will involve conscious processes of a more complex nature. I would not be surprised if, when faced with situations that the individual truly and cognitively perceives as threatening, extreme hyperactivity of the amygdala is observed during this altered state of consciousness. Many people claim to have visited hell and been trapped there for the most eternal hours of their existence. Be careful!

We will close this section by reflecting on the long-term changes the functional organization of the brain goes through. Carhart-Harris's 2017 fMRI study on depressed patients that had undergone psilocybin-assisted therapy found two connectivity changes that predicted improvement in depressive symptoms at week five post treatment. And both involved the prefrontal cortex, an area of the motor lobe involved in determining which actions an individual should perform based on their identity. It is likely, however, that many more connectivity changes associated with symptom improvement are yet to be discovered, as in that study, only four a priori selected areas were explored. Frederick Barrett's team carried out a further analysis published in 2020 (not mentioned in the previous lines) in which they studied long-term connectivity changes across the whole brain and found that the overall connectivity of the brain increased significantly and that such changes were not limited to any particular functional network. It will therefore be interesting to explore in detail the connectivity changes of more areas. For example, how do changes in connectivity in the primary cortices relate to symptom improvement? Perhaps, now that the depressed person is not so absorbed in their inner world, they are more connected to executive areas of the frontoparietal network, reflecting greater processing of sensory information. I'm sure we'll have more answers soon!

Corporal Effects

Another component of the psychedelic experience that is less explored, but in my opinion fundamental, is the bodily component. Several things happen at this level.

To begin with, in this state, information from the body is distorted, making it difficult to recognize common physiological signals such as the need to go to the toilet or to drink water. You suddenly start to feel a certain discomfort, but it takes longer than usual to work out why. "Am I maybe cold? Or may I, instead, be thirsty?" one might think. And believe me when I tell you that you will have never experienced the joy of finally getting this need satisfied. What a tremendous wonder and what a fantastic pleasure you will feel as strange sounds of happiness and amazement most probably emerge from your being.

I believe that this builds a greater appreciation for the well-being of every day and, arguably, one of the most important foundations of happiness: gratitude (how nice it feels to be well!). One now becomes an easy prey to fits of healthy laughter, and, isn't laughter the best antidote to fear? After all, with every laugh a piece of existential stress is released, preventing it from building up to a point where it can crush us.

The psychedelic state is also a dissociative state in which the feeling of being in control of one's actions, that is, of being the agent that directs the body (and also the mind), is affected. Rather, things seem to happen through oneself, as if they were happening to us. You just have to disinhibit yourself and let yourself be carried away by something internal that seems to precede reason and logical thinking. Something that pulls you from "doing" mode, so developed in human beings, to "being" mode. To the here and now.

When studying the executive effects, we already commented on how in this "here and now" attention is not imaginatively solving any problems. There is no hurry to get anywhere, neither physically nor mentally. Rather, attention becomes trapped by the stimuli present within the experience. Many of these come from the body itself, both from the somatosensory cortex (what an incredible world of tactile sensations!) and from the insula, which monitors visceral information and breathing, making the rhythm of the latter (that rhythm that always accompanies us but which we tend to ignore), the rudder of the experience.

As with the other senses, bodily sensations are amplified, allowing us to connect with the body in a way that makes us more aware of what it feels. Whereas in ordinary states of consciousness one largely feels through the mental narrative that the ego generates, the same is not true in the psychedelic experience. In ordinary states one becomes the victim of one's own story, bursting into tears while an inner voice says: "Why does this have to happen to me? Why can't I get [insert here that which the ego *desires*]?" Instead, rather than mental, during the psychedelic experience, our feelings are highly embodied and important emotional information seems to manifest somatically,[31] which is why somatic therapies that aim to release energetic blockages in the body seem to combine very well with psychedelic-assisted therapy.

I have not yet had the chance to explore this theoretical field in depth. What I do know is that, if one allows it, a state in which the body takes control of itself (known in the ayurvedic medicine of the yogis as "the awakening of the kundalini") can occur. According to these traditions, kundalini is a life force that, until it awakens, remains coiled like a snake at the base of the spine. When awakened, it rises through the central axis of your body and exits at the crown of your head, releasing the energy blockages and regenerating you in the process. Claudio Naranjo, a pioneering psychiatrist in linking spiritual traditions to psychotherapy, discusses how the psychedelic experience promotes this spiritual phenomenon. According to him, we possess an energetic armor that, to maintain the body as always ready for action, inhibits its spontaneous activity. When during the psychedelic experience (and more generally during the spiritual experience) the ego weakens, the inhibition it exerts on the body relaxes, causing involuntary but orderly movements that, like waves, run from the feet to the head.

---

31. Soma means body. If something is expressed somatically, it means that it is expressed through the body. For example, accumulated psychic discomfort can be somatized. That is, it can begin to manifest through the body and give rise to physical discomfort.

In spiritual traditions, this has been expressed cross-culturally as a serpentine power through which the movement of an energetic life force, known to the yogis as *prana*, or as *chi* in traditional Chinese medicine, can heal. And, without quite understanding how, it seems that this phenomenon can indeed promote long-term changes in people. In fact, its potency is such that cases have even been described in which it has triggered, like the psychedelic experience, psychotic breaks known as "kundalini accidents" in people who were not adequately prepared to deal with it.

The highly embodied quality of the psychedelic experience can also promote long-term changes in the way we relate to our bodies. For example, there are frequent reports of people who, after such experiences, change their diet or begin to take care of themselves in some other way.

I know, not only from my personal experience but also from the strong relationship between Eastern meditative practices and the psychedelic experience, that the perception of the breath can change significantly. And that this change can last over time, fading little by little depending on how hard we try, on a daily basis, to remember our ability to evoke that inner core of calm and wisdom that the psychedelic experience revealed to us.

It would be very interesting to study how this increased perception of breathing relates to the magnitude and duration of the therapeutic effects: do we, by experiencing each inhalation and exhalation more fully after the psychedelic experience, calm the narrative mind, which is always racing as it imagines possible future threats and goals? How do changes in breathing relate to the behavior of the limbic system and the individual's basal state of alertness? Does the autonomic system respond less reactively to environmental stimuli during that state of "afterglow"[32] that follows after a good psychedelic experience?

On leaving the INSIGHT[33] party in 2021, I mentioned this idea to Drummond McCulloch, a Ph.D. fellow from Copenhagen University

---

32. Within the psychedelic community, the state of afterglow refers to the state of good mood that sometimes follows a psychedelic experience, which shares some similarity with a state of enlightenment.

33. INSIGHT is a conference in Berlin organized by the MIND Foundation that brings together hundreds of psychedelic researchers.

Hospital, who told me that in his next experiment he was going to explore precisely this body-brain-mind relationship, using a breathing task inside the functional MRI scanner the days following the psychedelic session. Let's hope the results come out soon!

The increased connection to the body could also play an important role in driving a change in self-destructive behaviors, especially in cases of addictions or anorexia nervosa, where the patient is physically damaging that part of him or herself. In this deconstructed state, the functions carried out by that bizarre sheath that accompanies us in life are no longer taken for granted, and instead, deep gratitude emerges for what is now, during the psychedelic session, being perceived as the sacred temple of our consciousness. Imagine the sense of guilt and regret when realizing the damage that, through the poor actions and decisions made under the shadow of the ego, we have inflicted upon the precious gift of our body that has been bestowed upon us! The result? An urgent need to apologize for the contempt and mistreatment inflicted upon one's body and, at last, the determination required to change the harmful behavior.

How psychedelics modify the perception of one's body, both its internal states and its place in the world, is at the moment, in my opinion, one of the most interesting and unexplored themes within the field, but a study led by Katrin Preller in 2018 has found some interesting results related to the connectivity of the somatic-sensory-motor cortex.

Recall that the primary somatosensory cortex and the primary motor cortex work together forming the somatic-sensory-motor network, the former receiving information from the skin, and the latter activating the muscles required to execute the action selected in the prefrontal cortex that we are going to carry out. Wilder Penfield, an American neurosurgeon in the 1960s, discovered that in the primary cortices of this network, information about the body is distributed topographically (i.e., forming a map). The illustration of this map has been called "Penfield's homunculus" and you can find an example in figure 43.

Preller's study mentioned above explored the global connectivity of the brain and found that, during the psychedelic experience, the degree to which the connectivity of the somatic-sensory-motor network to the rest of the brain increased, correlated with the intensity of the experience.

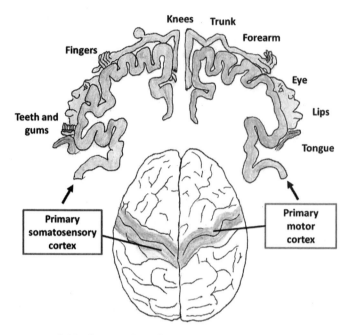

Figure 43. Penfield's homunculus of the somatic-sensory-motor cortex, showing in which areas of the cortex information from different parts of the body is represented (only some parts of the body are named). (See also color plate 20.)

But with what aspects of the experience exactly? Using a questionnaire designed to measure altered states of consciousness, the researchers found that the connectivity of this network was not only correlated with bodily aspects, such as the perceived degree of disembodiment (i.e., dissociation), but was also strongly correlated with the intensity of spiritual, visual, and semantic effects, as well as with feelings of joy and happiness.

If we focus on Yeo's parcellation of functional networks, the somatic-sensory-motor cortex is considered part of one of the primary nonassociative networks. Why might its behavior be so closely related to changes in higher functions? Perhaps this reminds you of the possible bodily component (in contrast to the narrative one) associated with ego dissolution that Alexander Lebedev spoke of in his 2015 study when he found that the disintegration of the salience network from Yeo's parcellation (i.e., the ventral attention network in figure 28 that contains the insula, a key interoceptive brain structure) was correlated with the magnitude of ego-dissolution.

Recall that in this study, researchers carried out an additional method of parcellation to the one performed by Yeo's team, and that in the parcellation performed by Lebedev's team[34] the somatic-sensory-motor cortex belonged to the same functional community as the insula. Finally, let us also recall that the study in 2016 led by Tagliazucchi and Roseman looking at changes in global connectivity found that ego dissolution was correlated to changes in insula connectivity. Perhaps this close relationship between the insula and the somatic-sensory-motor cortex explains why changes in the latter were so closely associated with changes in high-order functions in Preller's 2018 study. Could the connectivity of this area be reflecting the degree of disinhibition of the body armor described by Claudio Naranjo? Does such disinhibition not depend on ego dissolution? It will be interesting to study in the future how the changes in the somatic-sensory-motor cortex relate to the bodily movements associated with the kundalini awakening.

Finally, recall that the insula (working closely with the anterior cingulate cortex) is heavily involved in monitoring one's breathing. Martha Havenith, a research group leader at Ernst-Strüngmann Institute for Neuroscience and a breathwork facilitator has studied how, cross-culturally, multiple breathing techniques have been independently developed to access altered states of consciousness. One example is the technique developed to awaken the kundalini. Another is that of holotropic breathwork, a breathing technique consisting of accelerated breathing developed after LSD got banned by transpersonal psychologists Stanislav and Cristina Grof, who used it to access psychedelic-like highs and who have since trained and certified many facilitators. Finally, it should be remembered that during the psychedelic experience, breathing gains tremendous prominence and the usual breathing patterns change. It will therefore be interesting to study in more detail this close and fascinating relationship between the breath, the insula, the dissolution of the ego, the body armor, and the long-term changes

---

34. Yeo's parcellation of brain networks can be found in figure 28 of chapter 1.

in the body-mind relationship. I hope to have some answers for you in future publications! And of course, many more questions!

Unveiling the Psychedelic Experience's Transformative Potential

Having read this chapter, you will appreciate how the psychedelic experience produces profound changes in the behavior of the brain. Highly associative networks, such as the default mode network, the frontoparietal network, and the ventral attentional network, disintegrate, unleashing spontaneous activity in the medial temporal lobe. And at the same time as this area disconnects from these associative areas, its connection to the visual and somatosensory cortices increases, also increasing the dominance of these signals over brain activity. All this facilitates access to highly emotional and autobiographical material buried deep in the subconscious, giving the psychedelic experience a dreamlike quality full of amazing "visuals" and bodily sensations.

Attention is captured by the information available in the present moment while everything we have learned throughout our lives is questioned. Who are we? Why do we behave the way we do? And, above all, what is it that truly matters to us? This facilitates a reorganization of the relevance landscape within us that ultimately enables a change in our behavior.

Could it also be that as the belief of who we are is weakened, the anxiety triggered by the fear of not achieving the goals our ego desires is reduced? After all, many sages, including the Buddha, have postulated that desire is the source of all suffering and emphasized the vital importance of knowing how to accept and appreciate what we already do have.

During the psychedelic experience, the categorical separation between oneself and the outside world disappears. And as this happens, the inherent interconnectedness of everything around us becomes apparent with the utmost clarity. You are me and I am you. Let us take care of each other. We also cease to take for granted all the well-being and joy we have access to on a daily basis, awakening deep feelings of gratitude toward our bodies and toward existence on this dear Mother Earth, which every day provides us with light, air, water, food, and infinite beauty.

Although it is difficult and risky to establish a directionality between the different aspects of the experience, my personal interpretation is that such learned (or rather remembered) gratitude, acceptance, and connection defeats anxiety. From this newly found state of peace emerge feelings of self-compassion and love for oneself and others, thus increasing the likelihood of finally blossoming as one realizes one's full potential and moves toward it (which is the inherent desire of every living being) while wisely laughing in the face of this astounding cosmic joke called life.

Summary Tables of Studies

VISUAL EFFECTS			
Study	State	Object of Study	Results
Carhart-Harris (2016)	Resting-state (fMRI)*	Connectivity of VI (Primary visual (fMRI)* area)	Increased connectivity of VI with the rest of the brain.
Alamia and Timmermann (2020)	Resting-state (fMRI)*	Ascending and descending from the visual cortex.	Ascending waves increase and descending waves decrease.
Timmermann (2019)	Resting-state (EEG)	1. Brain waves 2. Complexity 3. Relationship between measures	1A. Collapse of alpha (midline) correlated with the intensity of the experience. 1B. Increased theta/delta (medial temporal lobe) correlated with the intensity of the experience. 2. Increased complexity (more pronounced in the occipital lobe) correlated with the intensity of the experience. 3A. Higher alpha collapse related to higher complexity. 3B. Higher alpha collapse related to higher delta/theta.

SEMANTIC EFFECTS (DISSOLUTION OF THE EGO)

Study	State	Object of Study	Results
Carhart-Harris (2014)	Resting during the psychedelic experience. EEG and fMRI	1. Brain waves (MEG) 2. Connectivity of the medial prefrontal cortex (fMRI) 3. Connectivity of the parahippocampal cortex (fMRI)	1. Reduced alpha waves in the posterior cingulate cortex are correlated with ego dissolution (Muthukumaraswamy et al, 2013). 2. Reduced connectivity between the medial prefrontal cortex and the posterior cingulate cortex. 3. Reduced connectivity between the parahippocampal cortex and posterior cingulate cortex correlated with ego dissolution.
Lebedev (2015)	Resting during the psychedelic experience. (fMRI)*	1. Global connectivity** 2. Yeo Networks 3. Alternative brain parcellation to the Yeo Networks	1. Medial temporal lobe disconnection with associative cortex correlates with ego dissolution. 2. The disintegration of the ventral attentional network described by Yeo, which contains the insula, correlates with ego-dissolution's intensity. 3. The insula belongs to the same functional community as the somatic-sensory-motor cortex.
Tagliazucchi and Roseman (2016)	Resting during the psychedelic experience. (fMRI)*	Global connectivity**	Connectivity changes in the insula are correlated with the dissolution of the ego. Changes in the connectivity of the angular gyrus are correlated with the dissolution of the ego.

SEMANTIC EFFECTS (DISSOLUTION OF THE EGO) (CONT'D)

Study	State	Object of Study	Results
Smigielski (2019)	Open-focus meditation on the day after the psychedelic experience. (fMRI)*	Connectivity of the medial prefrontal cortex	Reduced connectivity between the medial prefrontal cortex and the posterior cingulate cortex during open focus meditation correlates with the intensity of ego dissolution experienced during the psychedelic experience.

EXECUTIVE EFFECTS

Study	State	Object of Study	Results
Carhart-Harris (2014)	Resting-state (fMRI)*	Connectivity of the dorsolateral prefrontal cortex of the frontoparietal network	Disconnection between frontal and parietal areas of the frontoparietal executive network.

MNEMONIC EFFECTS

Study	State	Object of Study	Results
Carhart-Harris (2012)	Autobiographical recollection task (fMRI)*	Differences in brain activity during autobiographical memory recollection	1. There is no increased activity in the parahippocampal areas during psilocybin-induced recollection. 2. Increased activity in visual and somatosensory areas.

MNEMONIC EFFECTS (CONT'D)

Study	State	Object of Study	Results
Kaelen (2016)	Resting with music (fMRI)*	Medial temporal lobe connectivity	Increased connectivity with the visual cortex, correlated with the intensity of visuals of an autobiographical nature.
Timmermann (2019)	Resting-state (EEG)	Brain waves	Increased theta/ delta waves, possibly originating in the medial temporal lobe, correlated with the intensity of the experience.

EMOTIONAL REGULATION EFFECTS

Study	Population	Moment	Task	Results
Roseman (2019)	Not a clear selection (online study)	1. Two weeks before the experience and two weeks after the experience 2. Day after	1. Well-being questionnaires 2. Questionnaire on emotional content during the experience.	Psychedelics promote emotional experiences. The intensity of emotional experience correlates with improved well-being.
Kometer (2012)	Healthy (EEG)	During the psychedelic session	Reacting to positive or negative words	Greater reduction in the magnitude of the P300 for negative words than for positive words.
Mueller (2017)	Healthy (fMRI)*	During the psychedelic session	Reacting to facial expressions	Lower amygdala reactivity to negative faces correlated with higher intensity of the subjective effect.

EMOTIONAL REGULATION EFFECTS (CONT'D)				
Study	Population	Moment	Task	Results
Kraehenman (2016)	Healthy (fMRI)*	During the psychedelic session	Reacting to facial expressions	1. Lower amygdala reactivity to negative faces correlated with better mood at the end of the session. 2. Psilocybin affects the regulation of the amygdala over the visual cortex.
Grimm (2017)	Healthy (fMRI)*	During the psychedelic session	Reacting to facial expressions	Decreased connectivity between the amygdala and prefrontal cortex correlated with improved mood.
Preller (2015)	Healthy (fMRI)*	During the psychedelic session	Cyberball (social exclusion task)	Reduced sense of exclusion. Decreased activity in the anterior cingulate cortex correlated with the feeling of unity perceived during the experience.
Bershad (2020)	Healthy (fMRI)*	Under the effects of a microdose of LSD	Resting-state	Increased connectivity between the amygdala and the prefrontal cortex correlated with better mood.
Barrett (2020)	Healthy (fMRI)*	One week after the experience	1. Reacting to facial expressions 2. Task with conflicting emotional stimuli 3. Long-term changes in global connectivity	1. Reduced reactivity of the amygdala to negative stimuli. 2. Increased activity in the orbitofrontal cortex during the conflict task. 3. Increased global connectivity that is not limited to any particular functional network.

EMOTIONAL REGULATION EFFECTS (CONT'D)

Study	Population	Moment	Task	Results
Roseman (2018)	Depressed (fMRI)*	Day after the psychedelic session	Reacting to facial expressions	Increased amygdala reactivity to positive and negative stimuli.
Carhart-Harris (2017)	Depressed (fMRI)*	Day after the psychedelic session	Resting state	1. Reduced basal amygdala activity correlated with clinical symptoms. 2. No change in amygdala connectivity. 3. Improvement in clinical symptoms at five weeks is related to: a. Reduced connectivity between the parahippocampal cortex and the prefrontal cortex. b. Increased connectivity between the ventromedial prefrontal cortex and the angular gyrus.

BODILY EFFECTS

Study	State	Object of Study	Results
Preller (2018)	Resting during the psychedelic experience (fMRI)*	Global connectivity**	Increased connectivity between the somatic-sensory-motor cortex correlates with the intensity of the experience.

*fMRI: Functional Magnetic Resonance Imaging

**The three fMRI studies addressing global connectivity employed different analyses.

References for Further Study

Aqil M, Roseman L. 2023. More than meets the eye: the role of sensory dimensions in psychedelic brain dynamics, experience, and therapeutics. Neuropharmacology 223:109300.

Alamia A, Timmermann C, Nutt DJ, VanRullen R, Carhart-Harris RL. 2020. DMT alters cortical travelling waves. Elife 9:e59784.

Alexander BK. 2015. Healing addiction through community: A much longer road than it seems. Creating Caring Communities Conference.

Baggott MJ. 2015. Psychedelics and creativity: a review of the quantitative literature. PeerJ PrePrints 3:e1202v1.

Barrett FS, Doss MK, Sepeda ND, Pekar JJ, Griffiths RR. 2020. Emotions and brain function are altered up to one month after a single high dose of psilocybin. Scientific Reports 10(1):1–14.

Bershad AK, Preller KH, Lee R, Keedy S, Wren-Jarvis J, Bremmer MP, de Wit H. 2020. Preliminary report on the effects of a low dose of LSD on resting-state amygdala functional connectivity. Biological Psychiatry: Cognitive Neuroscience and Neuroimaging 5(4):461–467.

Carhart-Harris RL, Leech R, Williams TM, Erritzoe D, Abbasi N, Bargiotas T, Fielding A, et al. 2012. Implications for psychedelic-assisted psychotherapy: functional magnetic resonance imaging study with psilocybin. The British Journal of Psychiatry 200(3):238–244.

Carhart-Harris RL, Wall MB, Erritzoe D, Kaelen M, Ferguson B, De Meer I, Tanner M, Bloomfield M, Williams TM, Bolstridge M, et al. 2014. The effect of acutely administered MDMA on subjective and BOLD-fMRI responses to favourite and worst autobiographical memories. International Journal of Neuropsychopharmacology 17(4):527–540.

Carhart-Harris RL, Leech R, Hellyer PJ, Shanahan M, Feilding A, Tagliazucchi E, Chialvo DR, Nutt D. 2014. The entropic brain: a theory of conscious states informed by neuroimaging research with psychedelic drugs. Frontiers in Human Neuroscience 8:20.

Carhart-Harris RL, Muthukumaraswamy S, Roseman L, Kaelen M, Droog W, Murphy K, Tagliazucchi E, Schenberg EE, Nest T, Orban C, et al. 2016. Neural correlates of the LSD experience revealed by multimodal neuroimaging. Proceedings of the National Academy of Sciences USA 113(17):4853–4858.

Carhart-Harris RL, Roseman L, Bolstridge M, Demetriou L, Pannekoek JN, Wall MB, Tanner M, Kaelen M, McGonigle J, Murphy K, et al. 2017. Psilocybin for treatment-resistant depression: fMRI-measured brain mechanisms. Scientific Reports 7(1):1–11.

Fadiman J. 2011. The psychedelic explorer's guide: Safe, therapeutic, and sacred journeys. New York (NY): Simon & Schuster.

Family N, Vinson D, Vigliocco G, Kaelen M, Bolstridge M, Nutt DJ, Carhart-Harris RL. 2016. Semantic activation in LSD: evidence from picture naming. Language, Cognition and Neuroscience 31(10):1320–1327.

Grimm O, Kraehenmann R, Preller KH, Seifritz E, Vollenweider FX. 2018. Psilocybin modulates functional connectivity of the amygdala during emotional face discrimination. European Neuropsychopharmacology 28(6):691–700.

Hubbard EM, Ramachandran VS. 2005. Neurocognitive mechanisms of synesthesia. Neuron 48(3):509–520.

Kaelen M, Roseman L, Kahan J, Santos-Ribeiro A, Orban C, Lorenz R, Barrett FS, Bolstridge M, Williams T, Williams L, et al. 2016. LSD modulates music-induced imagery via changes in parahippocampal connectivity. European Neuropsychopharmacology 26(7):1099–1109.

Kometer M, Schmidt A, Bachmann R, Studerus E, Seifritz E, Vollenweider FX. 2012. Psilocybin biases facial recognition, goal-directed behavior, and mood state toward positive relative to negative emotions through different serotonergic subreceptors. Biological Psychiatry 72(11):898–906.

Kraehenmann R, Preller KH, Scheidegger M, Pokorny T, Bosch OG, Seifritz E, Vollenweider FX. 2015. Psilocybin-induced decrease in amygdala reactivity correlates with enhanced positive mood in healthy volunteers. Biological Psychiatry 78(8):572–581.

Kraehenmann R, Schmidt A, Friston K, Preller KH, Seifritz E, Vollenweider FX. 2016. The mixed serotonin receptor agonist psilocybin reduces threat-induced modulation of amygdala connectivity. NeuroImage: Clinical 11:53–60.

Lebedev AV, Lövdén M, Rosenthal G, Feilding A, Nutt DJ, Carhart-Harris RL. 2015. Finding the self by losing the self: Neural correlates of ego-dissolution under psilocybin. Human Brain Mapping 36(8):3137–3153.

Mason NL, Mischler E, Uthaug MV, Kuypers KP. 2019. Sub-acute effects of psilocybin on empathy, creative thinking, and subjective well-being. Journal of Psychoactive Drugs 51(2):123–134.

Mueller F, Lenz C, Dolder PC, Harder S, Schmid Y, Lang UE, Liechti ME, Borgwardt S. 2017. Acute effects of LSD on amygdala activity during processing of fearful stimuli in healthy subjects. Translational Psychiatry 7(4):e1084–e1084.

Muthukumaraswamy SD, Carhart-Harris RL, Moran RJ, Brookes MJ, Williams TM, Errtizoe D, Sessa B, Papadopoulos A, Bolstridge M, Singh KD, et al. 2013. Broadband cortical desynchronization underlies the human psychedelic state. Journal of Neuroscience 33(38):15171–83.

Naranjo C. 1996. The interpretation of psychedelic experience in light of the psychology of meditation. Sacred Plants, Consciousness and Healing 75–90.

Noorani T, Garcia-Romeu A, Swift TC, Griffiths RR, Johnson MW. 2018. Psychedelic therapy for smoking cessation: qualitative analysis of participant accounts. Journal of Psychopharmacology 32(7):756–769.

Preller KH, Pokorny T, Hock A, Kraehenmann R, Stämpfli P, Seifritz E, Scheidegger M, Vollenweider FX. 2016. Effects of serotonin 2A/1A receptor stimulation on social exclusion processing. Proceedings of the National Academy of Sciences USA 113(18):5119–5124.

Preller KH, Burt JB, Ji JL, Schleifer CH, Adkinson BD, Stämpfli P, Seifritz E, Repovs G, Krystal JH, Murray JD, et al. 2018. Changes in global and thalamic brain connectivity in LSD-induced altered states of consciousness are attributable to the 5-HT2A receptor. Elife 7:e35082.

Roseman L, Demetriou L, Wall MB, Nutt DJ, Carhart-Harris RL. 2018. Increased amygdala responses to emotional faces after psilocybin for treatment-resistant depression. Neuropharmacology 142:263–269.

Roseman L, Haijen E, Idialu-Ikato K, Kaelen M, Watts R. Carhart-Harris R. 2019. Emotional breakthrough and psychedelics: validation of the emotional breakthrough inventory. Journal of Psychopharmacology 33(9):1076–1087.

Smigielski L, Scheidegger M, Kometer M, Vollenweider FX. 2019. Psilocybin-assisted mindfulness training modulates self-consciousness and brain default mode network connectivity with lasting effects. NeuroImage 196:207–215.

Tagliazucchi E, Roseman L, Kaelen M, Orban C, Muthukumaraswamy SD, Murphy K, Laufs H, Leech R, McGonigle J, Crossley N, et al. 2016. Increased global functional connectivity correlates with LSD-induced ego dissolution. Current Biology 26(8):1043–1050.

Timmermann C, Roseman L, Schartner M, Milliere R, Williams LT, Erritzoe D, Muthukumaraswamy S, Ashton M, Bendrioua A, Kaur O, et al. 2019.

Neural correlates of the DMT experience assessed with multivariate EEG. Scientific Reports 9(1):1–13.

Watkins NW. 2018. (A)phantasia and severely deficient autobiographical memory: Scientific and personal perspectives. Cortex 105:41–52.

Watts R, Day C, Krzanowski J, Nutt D, Carhart-Harris R. 2017. Patients' accounts of increased "connectedness" and "acceptance" after psilocybin for treatment-resistant depression. Journal of Humanistic Psychology 57(5):520–564.

4

Psychedelic Neurobiology, Chaos, and Remodeling

Neurobiological Mechanisms of Action

In the previous chapter we looked at the subjective effects of psychedelics and changes in the intrinsic functional architecture of the brain, but how exactly do these molecules cause these changes? Why does the brain behave in this way and not another? What effects do these molecules have on neurons? And on which neurons specifically?

We are far from having all the answers. But we do have some. We know, for example, that psychedelics can bind to many different receptors on the membranes of neurons, but one is particularly important. After all the uncertainty of the previous chapter, I am glad to tell you that, thanks to some experiments, we now have no doubt about this. This was first demonstrated in humans by a study led by Vollenweider all the way back in 1998, when high doses of psilocybin were administered after ketanserin, a molecule that blocks a specific receptor, thus preventing the psychedelic substance from binding to it. The researchers found that under these circumstances the characteristic pychotomimetic effects of psilocybin did not occur, and further research led by Friederike Holze, from Matthias Liechti's team at the University of Basel, in 2021 demonstrated that ketanserin can also revert the acute response to LSD even when administered after the psychedelic. Ketanserin's ability to block psychedelic effects has not only been demonstrated through the use of questionnaires measuring participants' subjective experience. Several neuroimaging studies, such as a study in 2016 led by Katrin Preller revealed that ketanserin also blocks the functional connectivity changes promoted by psychedelics. At last, a definitive answer: the receptor blocked by ketanserin is certainly involved in the psychedelic experience! But which receptor is it, you may be asking yourself? It is a serotonin receptor: the 2A receptor.

Functioning of the Serotonin 2A Receptor

Since the serotonin 2A receptor appears to play a fundamental role in the psychedelic experience, it is pertinent to study it in more detail in order to understand how psychedelics cause the changes in brain behavior discussed in the previous chapter, or at least speculate about them more accurately. What is the function of the 2A receptor under normal conditions and what happens when, instead of serotonin, a psychedelic molecule attaches to it?

The first thing to know is that when serotonin binds to this particular receptor, it does not act as a neurotransmitter, but as a neuromodulator. Let me explain the difference. Neurotransmitters can produce an action potential by generating sharp, local currents of ions across the neuronal membrane, whereas neuromodulators do not cause action potentials, but rather, in a slower and more dispersed way, transform the interior of the neuron so that, when signals reach other receptors with neurotransmitter function, the neuron will fire more easily.

Let's take a closer look at exactly how the serotonin 2A receptor works. In short, under normal circumstances, stimulation of this receptor alone does not cause the firing of an action potential, but it does make the cell more likely to fire. How? Let's recall that for a neuron to fire an action potential, the amount of positive charge inside the neuron needs to surpass a certain threshold—namely, the threshold that causes the voltage-sensitive sodium channels in the axon to open and propagate the action potential through the membrane all the way down to the axon terminal. So, how does the serotonin 2A receptor facilitate the firing of action potentials? Recall that the cellular membrane is populated with various channels and that, depending on the signals the cell receives, these could be open or closed, allowing or preventing the passage of ions. To understand the workings of the serotonin 2A receptor we need to pay special attention to the potassium channels located in the membrane. Given that when the neuron is in its baseline state (called its resting potential) the concentration of potassium is much higher inside the neuron than outside, if the potassium channels are opened, potassium will exit the neuron following the concentration gradient (see the right side of figure 44). Because potassium is positively charged, its exit will reduce the positive charge inside the neuron, making it harder for the neuron to reach the threshold required to open the voltage-dependent sodium channels located in the axon that are responsible for the propagation of the action potential. Thus, one way of facilitating the firing of action potentials is to close the potassium channels in order to stop these positive ions from exiting the cell. This is precisely what serotonin does when it binds to the 2a receptors: it triggers a cascade of intracellular information that causes these potassium channels to close, and as a consequence potassium now begins to slowly accumulate inside the neuron (see figure 44). However, the accumulation of potassium ions inside the neuron due to the stimulation of the 2a receptor alone is not enough to trigger an action potential; it does, however, bring the neuron closer to being able to fire one, which is why we say that when serotonin binds to the 2a receptor it acts as a neuromodulator rather than as a neurotransmitter. This means that when the neuron then gets stimulated by excitatory neurotransmitters, if the 2a receptor has been previously stimulated, less amount of neurotransmitter will be required to get the neuron to fire an action potential and transfer the information to the next neuron. So basically, when serotonin binds to the 2a receptor it prepares the neuron for action but does not fire an action potential. This is the ingenious way in which this receptor, even without causing an action potential itself, exerts its excitatory function on neurons and partakes in the gating of information transfer throughout the brain.

How can one remain unmoved by the complex and beautiful informational dance inherent in every organism, all encoded in bioelectrical

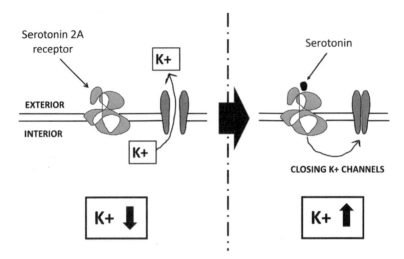

Figure 44. Functioning of the serotonin 2A receptor. When serotonin binds to this receptor, it causes potassium channels to close, promoting a progressive and diffuse increase in positive charge inside the neuron.

signals and the microscopic yet incommensurable DNA code? How can one not bow down before the ingenuity of Nature and the beautiful anarchic order that emerges from it at every scale? The pink sky coloring the sea at sunset, the perfect symmetry and grace of a passionflower, the interwoven wings of an electric dragonfly, the mesmerizing dance of birds of paradise, and so on. Beauty and complexity abound all around us, the product of the workings of a higher order whose rules we do not know, whatever they may be. The fantastic and magical potential of chance underlying natural selection!

After this brief moment of ecstasy, let's go back to the serotonin 2A receptor and how it is responsible for allowing psychedelic molecules to show us a new reality. What happens when instead of serotonin a psychedelic molecule binds to this receptor?

In vitro experiments (i.e., on cells grown in the laboratory) show that these molecules cause a spontaneous and excessive generation of action potentials in those neurons that contain 2A receptors in their membranes. Why might this be happening? What additional effect to that caused by serotonin could these molecules be having on the 2A receptor?

Inside the neuron, there is constant trafficking of receptors and in the cell membrane, a great fluidity: receptors being introduced or eliminated, and sometimes even forming heterodimers between them, i.e., two different receptors coming together and starting to work jointly. I did warn you at the beginning of the book about the infinite complexity we are facing! In the case of the serotonin 2A receptor, we know that it can form heterodimers with a glutamate receptor, mglu2. Unlike what happens after serotonin binds to the 2A receptor, when glutamate binds to the mglu2 receptor, it causes potassium channels to open. This facilitates the outflow of this ion and thus hinders the generation of an action potential, being one of the few glutamate receptors that have inhibitory rather than excitatory effects on the neuron (figure 45). The receptors that form this heterodimer are therefore antagonistic, since each one of them affects the total balance of charges inside the neuron in opposite directions.

Could it be then that the excessive neuronal activity caused by psychedelics is the result of their binding to the 2A receptor, causing the 2A receptor to inhibit the mglu2 receptor of this heterodimer? If the binding of psychedelics to the 2A receptor causes not only the closure

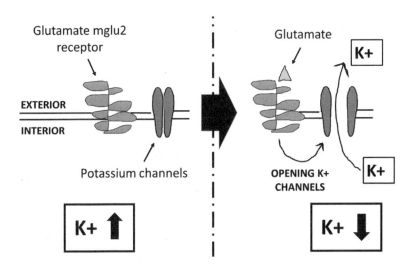

Figure 45. Functioning of the mglu2 receptor. When glutamate binds to this receptor, it causes potassium channels to open, decreasing the overall positive charge inside the neuron.

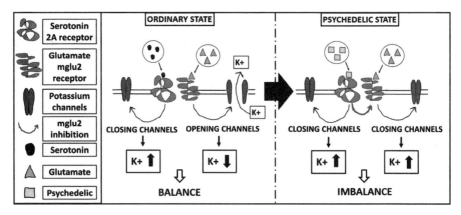

Figure 46. Function of the 2A-mglu2 heterodimer in ordinary states and under the action of a psychedelic. When, instead of serotonin, a psychedelic molecule binds to the 2A receptor, it inhibits the action of mglu2, producing an excessive accumulation of potassium in the interior of the neuron that causes a strong imbalance of charges, causing the spontaneous generation of action potentials.
(See also color plate 21.)

of potassium channels (as serotonin does) but also the inhibition of the mglu2 receptor that keeps them open, a rapid increase in potassium and positive charge inside the neuron should follow such binding, making the neuron fire much more easily, even spontaneously, as it happens in in vitro experiments (figure 46).

If this is how classic psychedelics alter neuronal behavior, what happens when they are administered together with a molecule that enhances the action of the mglu2 receptor? By counteracting the glutamate receptor inhibition promoted by the psychedelic molecule, the administration of molecules that promote mglu2 receptor activation should also eliminate the effects of psychedelics. A study in mice led by Michael A. Benneyworth in 2007 shows that this is in fact the case: when they administered a molecule that enhances mglu2 activation together with a psychedelic substance, it was observed that the head movements characteristic of the psychedelic state in mice did not appear. In other words, activating the mglu2 receptor seems to block the characteristic effects of psychedelic molecules, in the same way that the subjective effects in humans disappeared when researchers such as Vollenweider (1998), Preller (2016), or Holze (2021) blocked the serotonin 2A receptor with ketanserin. Benneyworth's results in mice, where activating the mglu2 receptor reverts the rodent's characteristic behavior under psychedelics, certainly support the 2A-mglu2 heterodimer theory, which postulates that psychedelic molecules promote the chaotic firing of neurons because of the particular way in which they activate the 2a receptor, leading to the inhibition of the mglu2 receptor, thus causing the positively charged potassium ion to rapidly accumulate inside the cell and uncontrollably fire action potentials. To reaffirm this mechanism of action in humans, it will be necessary to find molecules suitable for human consumption that potentiate the action of this glutamate receptor, in order to further replicate in humans the effects found in mice by Benneyworth, whereby stimulation of the mglu2 receptor (and thus opening of potassium channels) blocked psychedelic-related behavior.

Distribution of the Serotonin 2A Receptor

Be that as it may, there is no doubt that psychedelic molecules excessively increase the firing of 2A receptor-bearing neurons, but which neurons are they exactly? What is the distribution map of this neuromodulatory serotonin receptor?

Depending on which technique is used, slightly different distribution maps are obtained. And although they have several similarities, they also have striking differences, especially in relation to the density of this receptor in the visual cortex. For example, when using PET, a technique in which a radiopharmaceutical is administered, which is detectable by the scanner and which, without activating them, binds to 2A receptors located on neuronal membranes, the visual cortex does not appear to be the area with the highest density of these receptors (see the upper map in color plate 22[1]). However, when using a database for each brain area, containing the levels of messenger RNA associated with the protein that makes up the 2A receptor, the visual cortex does appear to

---

1. Image modified from the following article: Beliveau V, Ganz M, Feng L, Ozenne B, Højgaard L, Fisher PM, Svarer C, Greve DN, Knudsen GM. 2017. A high-resolution in vivo atlas of the human brain's serotonin system. Journal of Neuroscience 37(1):120–128.

be the area containing the greatest amount of this receptor (see lower map in color plate 22[2]).

Although there is, of course, a certain relationship between the levels of messenger RNA and the levels of the protein generated by this messenger RNA (i.e., the 2A receptor), this correlation is not as strong as one would expect, as can be seen in the differences between the two distribution maps. This may be due to several reasons, for example, because there is significant trafficking of receptors and messenger RNA within the neuron that is not detected by the PET technique. It is difficult to know which technique is more accurate. However, several studies have found that the distribution maps obtained using messenger RNA correlate with the magnitude of the connective disruption of each brain area during the psychedelic experience (the greater the amount of messenger RNA associated with the 2A protein, the greater the disruption), suggesting that the map obtained through messenger RNA is functionally informative.

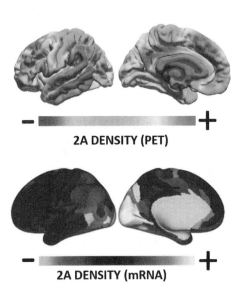

2A DENSITY (PET)

2A DENSITY (mRNA)

Figure 47. Serotonin 2A receptor distribution. *Above* is the distribution map of the 2A receptor using PET and *below* is the distribution map using messenger RNA (mRNA). The image *above* is modified from a study led by Beliveau and published in *The Journal of Neuroscience* in 2016. The *bottom* image was modified from a study led by Preller published in *eLife* in 2018. (See also color plate 22.)

---

2. Image modified from the following article: Preller KH, Burt JB, Ji JL, Schleifer CH, Adkinson BD, Stämpfli P, Seifritz E, Repovs G, Krystal JH, Murray JD, et al. 2018. Changes in global and thalamic brain connectivity in LSD-induced altered states of consciousness are attributable to the 5-HT2A receptor. Elife 7:e35082.

Whether or not the visual cortex is the area with the highest density of 2A receptors in its membranes, what is clear is that there is a significant amount of them in this brain region.

Let's continue comparing the distribution maps. Regardless of which technique is used, it seems that both seem to agree that the default mode network areas have a high density of these receptors, although you can see how this high receptor density is not limited to these areas alone. They also appear to be located extensively in other associative areas of the prefrontal and parietal cortex. No wonder these molecules seriously alter our ordinary state of consciousness!

As for the areas with lower 2A receptor levels, you can see how both maps show that these are not excessively abundant in the medial temporal lobe or the somatic-sensory-motor cortex, nor do they appear to be abundant in the insular cortex or the anterior part of the cingulate cortex. It is striking how, except for the angular gyrus, the different analyses employed to study global connectivity using functional magnetic resonance imaging have found that the intensity of the psychedelic experience was associated with the connective disruption in areas with low 2A receptor density: the medial temporal lobe in Lebedev's 2015 study, the insula in Tagliazucchi's and Roseman's 2016 study, and the somatic-sensory-motor cortex in Preller's 2018 study. What could this be due to?

Despite the great unknown that alpha waves still represent, we have already mentioned that the cognitive literature has associated them with processes involved in the suppression of the spontaneous activity of more primitive areas such as the hippocampal or visual areas, that is, with top-down processing. The appearance of these waves has also been associated with the medial areas of the default mode network, and we have seen that during the psychedelic experience these waves collapse. More specifically, remember that the magnitude of the collapse was correlated with the intensity of the experience in those signals collected from electrodes located over the posterior cingulate cortex. As can be seen in both distribution maps, the posterior cingulate cortex has a high density of 2A receptors. It is likely then that the collapse of the alpha waves is the consequence of the desynchronization that this area undergoes as the spontaneous activity of its neurons begins to increase. Recall that in 2019 a study from the Imperial College led by Timmermann found that the collapse of alpha waves was related to an increase in theta and delta waves (waves associated with the medial temporal lobe and REM sleep) and also to an increase in the complexity of signals from the visual cortex. He further found that the intensity of these two changes was also associated with the intensity of the experience, suggesting that the collapse of alpha may be triggering spontaneous activity in other areas (e.g. visual and hippocampal) and that the degree to which this happens determines the subjective effects promoted by psychedelics.

As we have discussed, except for the angular gyrus, all the results obtained through the study of global connectivity changes correlate the intensity of ego dissolution with the connective disruption of areas with low 2A receptor density. Given that the brain is hierarchically organized, with the default mode network possibly occupying the highest position in the hierarchy, it is most likely that the connectivity changes in these areas are the indirect effects of the disruption produced in the firing patterns of the higher-order areas, where these receptors are abundant. But why is it that it is the connective disruption in areas with low 2A receptor density (except for the angular gyrus) that best informs us about the intensity of the psychedelic experience? Could it perhaps be because the nature of these signals, and their changes, reflects, in an integrated manner, that which is happening in areas with high 2A receptor density?

Complex statistical methods will have to be employed to explore this interesting question in more detail. For example, what higher-order changes are associated with greater connective disruption of the insula or somatic-sensory-motor cortex? The fact that connective disruption of the angular gyrus during the psychedelic experience correlates with ego dissolution, combined with the fact that, after the experience, increased connectivity between this area and the ventromedial prefrontal cortex correlates with improvement in depressive symptoms, makes this a particularly interesting area on which to focus future studies. Is there a particular change in its connectivity that is influencing signaling from areas with low receptor density? A host of questions await answers!

Deep Cortical Layers, Chaos, and Belief Deconstruction

Having studied the distribution maps of this receptor, the next natural step is to delve into the cerebral cortex and study where these receptors are located within that structure. Remember that the cerebral cortex is organized horizontally in layers, and vertically in columns (figure 14 in chapter 1). Following the complex nature inherent to neuroscience, the fact is that these receptors appear on many cortical and subcortical neurons, but the dominant theories of psychedelic action pay particular attention to specific ones. Care to guess which? Remember perhaps those neurons in the deep layers of the cortex? It turns out that there is a high density of 2A receptors in their dendrites. This has a multitude of implications.

The first implication involves the mechanisms that the cortex employs to self-regulate through the control of thalamic activity. In figure 48 you can find an image combining figure 12 and 13, presented in

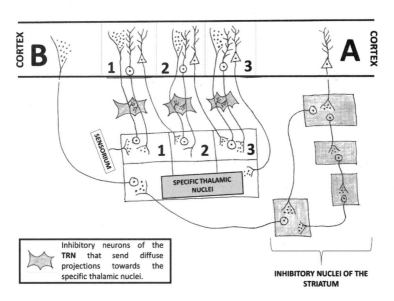

Figure 48. Cortical self-regulatory mechanisms through the control of the thalamic filter. The regulation of thalamic activity via inhibitory neurons in the TRN and the nuclei of the striatum is shown. These receive information from the cortex and modify the information it receives from the thalamus.

chapter 1 on neuroscience, where you can see how neurons in the deep layers send vertical projections to both the thalamic reticular nucleus and the striatum. Remember that both structures are composed of inhibitory neurons through which thalamic neurons are inhibited. In this way, these two structures regulate the thalamic information that ascends to the cortex, acting as a filter: the thalamic filter.

The spontaneous generation of action potentials by neurons in the deep layers will logically have a strong impact on the thalamic filter, producing significant changes in the information that the thalamus sends to the cortex. And, indeed, this change in the thalamic filter under psychedelics has been demonstrated by the 2018 study from Vollenweider's group led by Preller, using functional magnetic resonance imaging. This is probably a major mechanism underpinning the subjective effects contained within this extraordinary experience.

It is worth mentioning here that the neurons of the striatum and the thalamic reticular nucleus also have 2A receptors; hence the thalamic filter may be directly affected by psychedelics (i.e., independently of the pyramidal neurons of the cortex). Could, for example, the frequently experienced synesthesia be the result of psychedelics disorganizing the usual segregation of sensory information at the level of the thalamus? If the information here loses its usual segregation (due to changes in the neurons of the thalamic reticular nucleus responsible for coordinating the different thalamic nuclei), mixed sensory information could reach consciousness and give rise to the synesthetic phenomenon.

The fact that dendrites in the deep cortical layers have a high density of these receptors also has serious implications from the predictive coding point of view. Recall that, according to this theory, neurons in intracortical circuits:

1. Collect bottom-up information:
   a. from the thalamus
   b. from the prediction errors sent by the lower-order cortical columns, which carry an associated precision.
2. Collect top-down information:

a. from the predictions generated by the higher-order columns, which also carry an associated precision.

3. Calculate the prediction error between bottom-up and top-down information.

Recall also that, according to this theory, neurons in the deep layers encode, in their firing patterns, the information of the predictions made by each column, and that they send this information both vertically, to subcortical structures, and horizontally to the lower-order column.

If indeed, as this theory postulates, under normal conditions, the action potentials of these deep layer neurons contain information about the predictions being made by the model, this information will be logically affected by changes in their firing patterns. Consider the effects this will have on the prediction error computations. Recall that, according to this theory, each column calculates a prediction error by comparing the incoming information from the lower levels with the predictions made by the cortical columns at higher levels, and that it does this taking into consideration the accuracy associated with the incoming information and the descending prediction (see figure 15 from chapter 1). It is not hard to imagine the enormous impact that changing the firing patterns that encode the prediction made in level X+1 will have on the prediction error calculated at the X level! In these psychedelic circumstances, the higher-order columns will be unable to adequately predict the incoming information, consequently generating a multitude of prediction errors that, under normal conditions, would have been suppressed. The end result is an increase in bottom-up information and a decrease in the precision associated with the predictions.

Now recall the EEG study by Alamia and Timmermann at Imperial College London in 2020 measuring changes in ascending and descending waves under the effects of DMT. Could the predominance of ascending waves, detected in that study, be reflecting the increase in prediction errors generated by the informational disorganization of higher-order models? This is what the dominant theories centered around predictive coding would postulate. However, taking into consideration the high density of 2A receptors in the visual cortex, one could alternatively conjecture (as my friend Marco Aqil, the student I mentioned earlier, does) that the predominance of visual signals and the rise of visual information observed in the experiments is, at least in part, due to the direct stimulation that psychedelics are exerting on the 2A receptors located here. In other words, perhaps it is not just that the predictions of the associative areas are out of phase and, as they are unable to predict the incoming information, a greater number of prediction errors are generated. Perhaps more prediction errors are generated because the visual cortex is being stimulated in a novel way that is not contained in the expectations generated by the model. Similarly, the relationship found in 2019 by Timmermann between alpha-wave collapse and increased complexity in the signals of the visual cortex under the effects of DMT could perhaps be understood the other way around. The increase in the complexity of visual cortex signals might not be due to the collapse of alpha waves, but rather, the collapse of alpha waves might be due to the increased complexity of signals in the visual cortex caused by direct stimulation of the receptors that abound here. The two theories are not mutually exclusive, and the observed results could be due to a combination of the two.

Be that as it may, the bottom line is that, whereas in ordinary states of consciousness, whether or not the neurons fire is carefully determined by the set of information received by all the neurons' synapses (each with their respective strengths finely established and updated through experience), now the neurons in the deep cortical layers fire in a much more chaotic and spontaneous way. Or, as Andrew Gallimore, a neurobiologist, and DMT expert, would say, the connections between neurons are democratized. They are no longer so strongly determined by synaptic forces sculpted over the course of a lifetime, and the usual organization of the brain is lost. I would like to take this opportunity to encourage you to watch the extensive and entertaining course on psychedelic neuroscience that Gallimore has produced and uploaded to YouTube. It is an excellent work through which this eccentric character will make you laugh out loud while he guides you in detail through the workings of the psychedelic brain. Thank you, Gallimore, for so much information, for so many laughs, and for answering all my questions! You are an excellent communicator.

In short, in the psychedelic state, the usual intrinsic functional architecture of the brain is lost, and the brain's dynamics become more unpredictable. We could say that, while in normal states the energy of the system gravitates around "heavy" states, forming relatively stable energy structures that fluctuate in a relatively predictable way (i.e., connectivity patterns), during the psychedelic experience, these energy structures lose weight. By absorbing less energy, they allow it to flow more freely and to distribute itself around lighter structures, which inevitably increases the total number of possible structures and states. Metaphorically, we could say that the brain's energetic dynamics rebel against the established order, becoming more chaotic, as has been fantastically exposed through the anarchic brain or the entropic brain hypotheses presented by Imperial College's group in 2019 and 2014, respectively.

Although entropy is a complicated concept, which we will not go into in depth, we must understand it as the degree of predictability and complexity of a system. To understand this concept a little better, imagine for example a system consisting of two neurons. If these always generate the action potential together, the total number of states in which the system can be found will be less than if each of them generated action potentials independently, since, in the first case, the state of one of them limits the state in which the other is found, while in the second case there is no such limitation. Consider that the greater the number of states in which the system can find itself, the greater its complexity, and the harder it will be to predict its behavior. That is, as entropy increases, the system becomes more complex and therefore less predictable. Following this logic, the psychedelic state undoubtedly has higher entropy than the ordinary state of consciousness, as has been corroborated by several studies. Having read this chapter, we now know why: neurons with 2A receptors gain independence from what is dictated to them by the neurons with which they usually communicate! In figure 49 you can see an artistic representation I have made of this theory. Each spiral represents a possible state that the system could be in, and their respective sizes represent the weight associated with each one of them as if they were whirlpools. Deeper eddies will be more stable

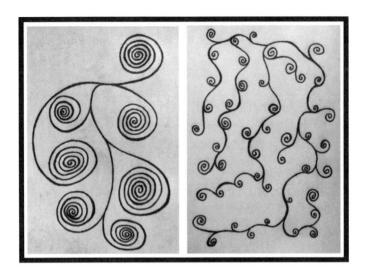

Figure 49. Artistic representation of an ordered brain (on the *left*) and a chaotic brain (on the *right*).

and will store more energy than lighter ones. As reflected in figure 49, in the ordinary state of consciousness, energy is distributed around a small number of deep eddies, whereas in the psychedelic state, the number of eddies increases, their being necessarily lighter. This new dynamic facilitates fluctuation between states, providing the system with flexibility. People trapped in a certain pattern of behavior or thinking will have extremely heavy and rigid structures.

When, with a high degree of confidence, we believe that we hold the answer to something, we do not question it and hence, don't generate alternative possibilities about that belief. As we consider fewer possibilities, fewer states will emerge that relate to the way we hold that belief. We have already seen that in the psychedelic state we, instead, question everything learned, dramatically increasing the number of possibilities associated with a given issue. This could be the reason why "magical" thinking, in which a person may begin to consider beliefs related to, for example, the ability of thoughts to influence the material world, or the possibility of a psychic reality independent of material reality often occurs during the psychedelic state. In this new ocean of psychedelic uncertainty, the opportunity to create a story increases, and, through such magical stories, we manage to reduce the uncertainty of the system just as we neuroscientists do when we try to interpret neuroimaging results!

Let us now imagine that each spiral in figure 49 represents a belief. Translating this into the language of predictive coding, we could say that the heaviness of the structure represents the degree of confidence (i.e., precision) with which the belief (i.e., prediction generated by the model) is held. For those beliefs held with high confidence, the synapses encoding the expectation will be strong, which will cause those synapses to be reinforced, making it even more difficult to revise them. It will take a strong perturbation to defeat this heavy structure and update the system. And that disruption is precisely what psychedelics seem to do.[3] By disrupting the information encoded in the synaptic forces associated with the belief, prediction errors that prior to the experience were being suppressed by the high confidence associated with it can finally be generated. The input of prediction errors also causes the system to lose confidence in the belief, thus facilitating its revision and the updating of the model.

This will not only allow us to detect occasional errors and biases in the cognitive or heuristic frameworks through which we process information. More generally, it will cause all beliefs, even those that are correct, to be held with less confidence, promoting greater open-mindedness. Beliefs are fragments of learned and integrated information that we use to work with and effectively determine how to respond to the information of a given moment. Certain stability in models of the world is necessary, as this is part of what learning is about: integrating and stabilizing important information for later use. However, having the ability to detect information that does not fit our model is key. Otherwise, we would not be able to update it. This is where having a certain degree of open-mindedness becomes essential. Without it, we run a great risk of ignoring important information.

And indeed, although the definition of personality refers to it as a structure that remains stable after the age of thirty, several studies have observed a lasting increase in the personality trait of open-mindedness

---

3. Electroconvulsive therapy used to treat severe depression may also work by generating such a disturbance. However, this therapy damages nerve tissue and does not promote moments of insight capable of restructuring beliefs in a way that is meaningful to the individual.

after a psychedelic experience. In 2018, a publication led by José Carlos Bouso presented a detailed review on how psychedelic substances affect personality structure in a way that appears to promote therapeutic effects. And another study from Imperial College led by Alexander Lebedev in 2016 even found that two weeks after a psychedelic experience, the increase in open-mindedness was correlated with the increase in brain entropy during the altered state of consciousness. Mind blowing how the energetic dynamics of the brain parallels the phenomenology of the experience and its consequences on personality structure!

Additionally, using laboratory tasks designed to measure cognitive flexibility, other studies have found it increases after a psychedelic experience. In these tasks, one has to follow a certain rule to solve the exercise, and this rule changes randomly. A classic test is the Wisconsin Card Sorting Test. Imagine a deck of cards. On each card, there is a certain geometrical figure (square, triangle, circle . . .), and the cards vary according to the number of figures on the card (e.g. three triangles) and according to the color of the figures (all figures on the card have the same color). Each time a card appears, you have to answer as quickly as possible according to the rule set at the time. One rule may be to answer according to the color of the card, another according to the number of figures on the card, and yet another according to the shape of the figure. For the researchers, this task aims to measure how well the participants adapt to the norm change when it happens: how fast do they adapt and how many mistakes do they make after the norm change? In this way, researchers measure some aspect of what we have called "cognitive flexibility," and this aspect seems to increase after a psychedelic experience.

A study in 2020 by Ashleigh Murphy-Beiner and Kirstie Soar measured this ability the day before and the day after an ayahuasca session in a group of forty-eight participants and found an increase in this measure, as well as an increase in people's perceived level of presence, as measured by a mindfulness questionnaire. Similarly, when four weeks after the psychedelic experience changes in cognitive flexibility were measured in the twenty-four depressed patients from Johns Hopkins's 2021 clinical trial on major depression, led by

Alan K. Davis, an increase in cognitive flexibility was also found. These behavioral analyses, led by Manoj Doss and published in 2021, did not find a correlation between symptom improvement and cognitive flexibility, but this could perfectly well be because the small number of participants did not allow for the possible therapeutic component of cognitive flexibility to be detected. After all, this increase is multifactorial. It could be, for example, that, through the experience, someone has increased their cognitive flexibility but has not managed to restructure their relevance maps. In other words, increased flexibility need not always be accompanied by profoundly revealing moments of insight that impact the individual. In short, although the study did not find a correlation between cognitive flexibility and symptom improvement, it would make sense that the increase in entropy during the experience, and the ensuing cognitive openness and flexibility, would be beneficial for people who are strongly susceptible to maladaptive beliefs or behaviors, since, by reducing the precision associated with beliefs, this entropic state would seem to promote greater flexibility and facilitate the updating of the system.

Neuroplasticity: Remodeling of the Mind and Brain

For this long-term updating of the system to occur, it is, of course, necessary that the cellular mechanisms underlying neuroplasticity are activated, and as my friend and neuroscientist Cato de Vos, in a collaboration with Natasha Mason and Kim Kuypers from Maastricht University, shows in a detailed literature review published in 2021, many studies have shown that psychedelics promote all the processes associated with this phenomenon: the creation of new synapses (i.e., synaptogenesis), the strengthening of old ones, the growth of dendrites and axons (neuritogenesis), and even the birth of new neurons (i.e., neurogenesis)! Let's look at some of the studies in more detail.

Remember for example the NMDA and AMPA glutamate receptors involved in reinforcing synaptic strengths that we studied when learning about neuroplasticity in chapter 1 (figure 4). A study from Federal University of Rio de Janeiro led by Vanja Dakic in 2017 has found an increase in these receptor proteins following a single dose of 5-MeO-DMT, a psychedelic obtained from the secretions of a Mexican Sonoran desert toad called *Bufo alvarius*. This study was conducted in vitro on human neurons and more specifically on human brain organoids.

Organoids are three-dimensional multicellular constructs that mimic the tissue in question, providing an advance over studying layers of neurons that have been dismembered from their surrounding tissue, as is often done in in vitro research. In another in vitro study in 2018 led by Calvin Ly, from the University of California, on neurons obtained from rat brains, they observed an increase in the complexity of dendritic arbors after applying both LSD and DMT to these neurons, with the effect being greater for LSD than for DMT, demonstrating that these molecules not only promote the strengthening of existing synapses, but also the creation of new ones.

As for neurogenesis, Jordi Riba, founder of the first psychedelic research group in Spain, was one of the world's pioneers in this field, studying, among other things, the neuroplastic properties of psychedelics. In addition to finding that the non-psychedelic component of the ayahuasca brew promoted neurogenesis, a future study in 2020 by Riba's team, led again by Jose A. Morales-García, demonstrated that the psychedelic component of ayahuasca, DMT, also promotes the proliferation of new neurons! In this study, neurons were again obtained from the hippocampal area of mice, where we know stem cells capable of becoming neurons reside, and after seven days of a daily DMT application, the researchers observed a significant proliferation of neurons. Moreover, this has been corroborated in in vivo experiments, both by this same team and by another team led by Lima da Cruz in 2018 using 5-MeO-DMT. In the latter study, they also implanted electrodes in mice's brains and directly measured their brain activity while they were alive. By doing this, they found that neurons fired more readily to stimuli after having received psychedelics, suggesting that synapse strengthening had occurred. This, of course, makes sense when we consider that in 2017 Dakic found an increase in AMPA- and NMDA-like proteins in the brain organoids. Nor is it surprising that when another in vivo study in rats from 2021, led by Oskar Hougaard Jefsen from

Aarhus University, looked at the composition inside prefrontal and hip-pocampal neurons ninety minutes after a dose of psilocybin had been administered, an increase in the expression of genes related to molecules involved in intracellular information cascades related to neuroplasticity was found.

Results from the in vitro literature go even further, showing that these molecules not only promote neuroplasticity, but they also appear to have neuroprotective properties! For example, a study led by Attila Szabo in 2016 subjected neurons to hypoxic stress (i.e., lack of oxygen) and observed a reduction in cell death when DMT was applied to them. These neuroprotective properties, however, are dose dependent and dis-appear at high doses, as shown for example by a study led by Albert Katchborian-Neto in 2020.

In human studies, neuroplasticity has been indirectly assessed by measuring the levels of BDNF in blood plasma. There are, however, only four studies and not all of them point in the same direction. For example, two studies have measured BDNF levels forty-eight hours after an ayahuasca session involving both healthy and depressed people, and while one study finds no increase in BDNF, the other study finds an increase in BDNF in both depressed and healthy people, even find-ing that, in depressed people, the increase in BDNF correlates with the decrease in depressive symptoms!

One possible explanation for this discrepancy is that this Amazonian cocktail does not consist of a strictly established recipe. Each commu-nity prepares it differently, and, depending on the specific purpose of the medicine at a given time, the composition may even vary within the same community. The different results could therefore be due to differences in the ayahuasca cocktail preparation. Finally, two studies have also found an increase of BDNF in the blood plasma within hours of consuming LSD.

How, then, do these molecules promote neuroplasticity? It seems that, like the subjective effects, neuroplasticity is also controlled by the serotonin 2A receptor, since when several of the studies used, along with the psychedelic, molecules that block the action of the 2A receptor, the observed neuroplastic effects disappeared. Neuroplastic processes involve complex intracellular cascades, and we know that the 2A receptor is, for example, responsible for regulating the cell's microtubules. Let's see what this means and why it is relevant.

Like animal bodies, the morphology of a neuron is supported by filamentous structures that act as a cellular skeleton (i.e., cytoskeleton).

These filaments are called microtubules and are made up of units called tubulins (figure 50). Depending on the information they receive, these units attach to or detach from the microtubule, lengthening or shortening it respectively. Through this dynamic process, the 2A receptor can modify the conformation of the neuron by stretching the neuronal body and, with it, the membrane. This allows new synaptic boutons to be generated in which to insert receptors and new dendrites and axons through which to transmit information. This fluidity in microtubule growth is particularly important in the processes of synaptogenesis and neuritogenesis.

This is just one of the processes through which neuroplasticity is promoted. We have also seen how synaptic reinforcement through AMPA and NMDA glutamate receptors is regulated by the amounts of glutamate present in the synaptic cleft (recall the information presented in figure 4). And psychedelics increase glutamate levels in the cortex, both directly and indirectly. Firstly, the binding of the psychedelic to neurons in deep cortical layers directly produces an increase in glutamate by causing the generation of spontaneous action potentials by

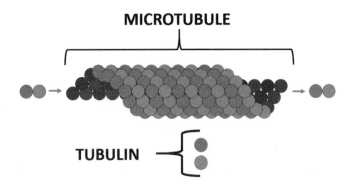

Figure 50. Diagram of a microtubule formed by tubulin proteins. Image obtained and modified from Simon Caulton. (See also color plate 23.)

these neurons. As we have seen when studying the theory of hierarchical predictive coding, the spontaneous firing of these deep-cortical neurons introduces noise into the top-down predictions, which in turn leads to the production of prediction errors, coded in the form of ascending action potentials thanks to the release of glutamate by the superficial levels of the cortex. The end result is a sharp increase in glutamate that could be reinforcing the strengthening of synapses in cortical neurons. It is not surprising then that Frederick Barrett and his team in 2020 found an increase in global connectivity when he assessed brain behavior a week after the psychedelic experience. After all, we have already seen how the distribution of 2A receptors is not limited to a single functional network.

Note also that neuroplasticity processes are highly involved in learning and are activated when new information is introduced into the system. It is not surprising then that these processes are activated during the psychedelic experience, given that, through the generation of prediction errors, the system is detecting a strong input of novel information that triggers the activation of all the neuronal mechanisms involved in learning.

Let us conclude with a metaphor presented by Robin Carhart-Harris and Karl Friston in 2019 in the theory of the anarchic brain. According to this metaphor, the effect psychedelics have on the architecture of the brain is equivalent to the effect of heat applied to metal in metallurgical techniques: they soften the rigidity of the structure, allowing it to take on a new shape as it cools.

The high state of neuroplasticity in which the associative areas are embedded during the psychedelic experience facilitates the new configuration of the brain to incorporate the information learned during the experience. And more specifically, could it be that the restructuring of long-term synaptic connections is being sculpted through the moments of insight experienced during the psychedelic trip?

In short, the relaxation of beliefs promoted in the psychedelic state, coupled with their high neuroplastic potential, makes these molecules powerful and useful tools capable of restructuring the relevance maps (possibly located in the most medial and ventral parts of the prefrontal cortex) that drive behavior, thought, emotions, and attention.

References for Further Study

de Almeida RN, de Menezes Galvão AC, Da Silva FS, Dos Santos Silva EA, Palhano-Fontes F, Maia-de-Oliveira JP, Barros de Araújo L-S, Lobão-Soares B, Galvão-Coelho NL. 2019. Modulation of serum brain-derived neurotrophic factor by a single dose of ayahuasca: observation from a randomized controlled trial. Frontiers in Psychology 10:1234.

Beliveau V, Ganz M, Feng L, Ozenne B, Højgaard L, Fisher PM, Svarer C, Greve DN, Knudsen GM. 2017. A high-resolution in vivo atlas of the human brain's serotonin system. Journal of Neuroscience 37(1):120–128.

Benneyworth MA, Xiang Z, Smith RL, Garcia EE, Conn PJ, Sanders-Bush E. 2007. A selective positive allosteric modulator of metabotropic glutamate receptor subtype 2 blocks a hallucinogenic drug model of psychosis. Molecular Pharmacology 72(2):477–484.

Bouso JC, Dos Santos RG, Alcázar-Córcoles MÁ, Hallak JE. 2018. Serotonergic psychedelics and personality: A systematic review of contemporary research. Neuroscience & Biobehavioral Reviews 87:118–132.

Carhart-Harris RL, Leech R, Hellyer PJ, Shanahan M, Feilding A, Tagliazucchi E, Chialvo DR, Nutt D. 2014. The entropic brain: a theory of conscious states informed by neuroimaging research with psychedelic drugs. Frontiers in human neuroscience 8:20.

Carhart-Harris RL, Friston K. 2019. REBUS and the anarchic brain: toward a unified model of the brain action of psychedelics. Pharmacological Reviews 71(3):316–344.

Dakic V, Minardi Nascimento J, Costa Sartore R, Maciel RDM, de Araujo DB, Ribeiro S, Martins-de-Souza D, Rehen SK. 2017. Short term changes in the proteome of human cerebral organoids induced by 5-MeO-DMT. Scientific Reports 7(1):1–13.

Davis AK, Barrett FS, Griffiths RR. 2020. Psychological flexibility mediates the relations between acute psychedelic effects and subjective decreases in depression and anxiety. Journal of Contextual Behavioral Science 15:39–45.

De Vos CM, Mason NL, Kuypers KP. 2021. Psychedelics and neuroplasticity: a systematic review unraveling the biological underpinnings of psychedelics. Frontiers in Psychiatry 1575.

Doss MK, Považan M, Rosenberg MD, Sepeda ND, Davis AK, Finan PH, Smith GS, Pekar JJ, Barker PB, Griffiths RR, et al. 2021. Psilocybin therapy increases cognitive and neural flexibility in patients with major depressive disorder. Translational Psychiatry 11(1):1–10.

Galvão-Coelho NL, de Menezes Galvão AC, de Almeida RN, Palhano-Fontes F, Campos Braga I, Lobão Soares B, Maia-de-Oliveira JP, Perkins D, Sarris J, Barros de Araujo D. 2020. Changes in inflammatory biomarkers are related to the antidepressant effects of ayahuasca. Journal of Psychopharmacology 34(10):1125–1133.

Holze F, Vizeli P, Ley L, Müller F, Dolder P, Stocker M, Duthaler U, Varghese N, Eckert A, Borgwardt S, et al. 2021. Acute dose-dependent effects of lysergic acid diethylamide in a double-blind placebo-controlled study in healthy subjects. Neuropsychopharmacology 46(3):537–544.

Hutten NR, Mason NL, Dolder PC, Theunissen EL, Holze F, Liechti ME, Varghese N, Eckert A, Feilding A, Ramaekers JG, et al. 2020. Low doses of LSD acutely increase BDNF blood plasma levels in healthy volunteers. ACS Pharmacology & Translational Science 4(2):461–466.

Jefsen OH, Elfving B, Wegener G, Müller HK. 2021. Transcriptional regulation in the rat prefrontal cortex and hippocampus after a single administration of psilocybin. Journal of Psychopharmacology 35(4):483–493.

Katchborian-Neto A, Santos WT, Nicácio KJ, Corrêa JO, Murgu M, Martins TM, Gomes DA, Goes AM, Soares MG, Dias DF, et al. 2020. Neuroprotective potential of Ayahuasca and untargeted metabolomics analyses: applicability to Parkinson's disease. Journal of Ethnopharmacology 255:112743.

Lebedev AV, Kaelen M, Lövdén M, Nilsson J, Feilding A, Nutt DJ, Carhart-Harris RL. 2016. LSD-induced entropic brain activity predicts subsequent personality change. Human Brain Mapping 37(9):3203–3213.

Lima da Cruz, RV, Moulin TC, Petiz LL, Leão RN. 2018. A single dose of 5-MeO-DMT stimulates cell proliferation, neuronal survivability, morpho-logical and functional changes in adult mice ventral dentate gyrus. Frontiers in Molecular Neuroscience 11:312.

Ly C, Greb AC, Cameron LP, Wong JM, Barragan EV, Wilson PC, Burbach KF, Zarandi SS, Sood A, Paddy MR, et al. 2018. Psychedelics promote structural and functional neural plasticity. Cell Reports 23(11):3170–3182.

Morales-Garcia JA, Calleja-Conde J, Lopez-Moreno JA, Alonso-Gil S, Sanz-SanCristobal M, Riba J, Perez-Castillo A. 2020. N,N-dimethyltryptamine compound found in the hallucinogenic tea ayahuasca, regulates adult neu-rogenesis in vitro and in vivo. Translational Psychiatry 10(1):1–14.

Murphy-Beiner A, Soar K. 2020. Ayahuasca's 'afterglow': improved mindfulness and cognitive flexibility in ayahuasca drinkers. Psychopharmacology 237(4):1161–1169.

Preller KH, Herdener M, Pokorny T, Planzer A, Kraehenmann R, Stämpfli P, Liechti ME, Seifritz E, Vollenweider FX. 2017. The fabric of meaning and subjective effects in LSD-induced states depend on serotonin 2A receptor activation. Current Biology 27(3):451–457.

Preller KH, Burt JB, Ji JL, Schleifer CH, Adkinson BD, Stämpfli P, Seifritz E, Repovs G, Krystal JH, Murray JD, et al. 2018. Changes in global and thalamic brain connectivity in LSD-induced altered states of consciousness are attributable to the 5-HT2A receptor. Elife 7:e35082.

Szabo A, Kovacs A, Riba J, Djurovic S, Rajnavolgyi E, Frecska E. 2016. The endogenous hallucinogen and trace amine N,N-dimethyltryptamine (DMT) displays potent protective effects against hypoxia via sigma-1 receptor activation in human primary iPSC-derived cortical neurons and microglia-like immune cells. Frontiers in Neuroscience 10:423.

Vollenweider FX, Vollenweider-Scherpenhuyzen MF, Babler A, Vogel H, Hell D. 1998. Psilocybin induces schizophrenia-like psychosis in humans via a serotonin-2 agonist action. Neuroreport 9:3897–3902.

5

MDMA: Love Enhancer, Fear Suppressor

In this chapter we will learn about MDMA's subjective and behavioral effects. We will also study how this molecule interacts with the nervous system and why all these effects might be therapeutic for people suffering from post-traumatic stress disorder, social anxiety and, even, alcoholism. But, what exactly is MDMA?

MDMA stands for 3,4-methylenedioxymethamphetamine, and its chemical structure resembles both that of stimulants (e.g., cocaine and amphetamines) and that of classic psychedelics. How does MDMA's phenomenology compare to theirs?

Phenomenology of MDMA: Feeling Safe

Compared to other stimulant drugs such as cocaine, MDMA does have a certain capacity to promote aspects of the mystical experience such as feelings of oneness, ineffability, blissfulness, gratitude, and even, ego dissolution. However, it is far from doing so with the intensity that classic psychedelics do. For example, a study led by Friederike Holze in 2020 shows how, under MDMA, of all the aspects of the mystical experience, only the intensity of blissfulness approaches that caused by classic psychedelics such as LSD. To investigate this, they used several questionnaires designed to measure the mystical experience and compared the abilities of placebo, amphetamine, MDMA, and LSD to promote different aspects of the experience. When studying these questionnaires, higher scores were obtained for MDMA than for placebo or amphetamine. However, except for blissfulness, the intensity of all remaining aspects of the experience was much lower for MDMA than for LSD. The same was true for visual and perceptual distortions. MDMA can certainly promote certain effects of this type, but not nearly as intensely as LSD, psilocybin, or DMT.

There are additional phenomenological reasons why MDMA is not a classic psychedelic. Fundamentally, MDMA does not affect the way in which thought unfolds; neither does it deconstruct the semantic network, nor does it affect the perception of time. For example, when Holze's study asked participants about changes in the speed of their thinking, only LSD seemed to affect this measure, seemingly slowing it down. As we saw in the previous chapters, it is assumed that the profound ego dissolution promoted by classic psychedelics is, at least in part, the product of the general deconstruction of meanings, something that does not happen under MDMA.

It is, therefore, possible that the ego-dissolution reported under both substances differs not only quantitatively, but also qualitatively. In addition, MDMA pushes the individual toward extroversion, whereas psychedelics pushes them toward introversion. This is why MDMA sessions consist of both periods of talk therapy and periods of silence and introspection, whereas sessions with classic psychedelics are mainly focused on the inward journey.

For all these reasons, some drug classifications have referred to substances such as MDMA as "pseudo-psychedelics." However, other classifications have preferred to focus on its main feature: its powerful impact on social aspects of behavior. This molecule generates a highly empathic emotional warmth. Because of this, in 1983, Ralph Metzner and David Nichols named these molecules "empathogens."

This ability to increase empathy has been demonstrated not only through the personal statements of consumers. Laboratory tasks have also been used. In these, it is common to present the participants with photos of people's faces showing strong emotional expressions and, during the task, ask them questions related to the emotions presented on the screen. Depending on the specific question, we can measure different aspects of empathy. For example, cognitive empathy can be captured through questions aimed at measuring the participant's understanding of the other's emotions (e.g., "How do you think the person in the picture is feeling?") But empathy is more than knowing or understanding another's emotional state. Empathy is a feeling. It is an emotion, and this aspect of empathy (i.e., emotional empathy) is measured with questions such as: "On a scale from 1 to 9, how much does the emotion of the person in the photo make you feel?" The difference between cognitive empathy and emotional empathy is well represented in psychopaths and sociopaths. These people have no problem in cognitively understanding the emotional state of people. In fact, some are particularly good at it, something that they use to manipulate others. But the same is not true when measuring emotional empathy. In this case, psychopaths and sociopaths demonstrate a severe inability to feel and identify with the other person's emotional state.

What happens then when this task is used to measure empathy under the effects of MDMA in healthy people? The results of several studies, such as one led by Kim Kuypers, seem to indicate that, although this molecule does not have a significant effect on cognitive empathy, it does have a significant effect on emotional empathy. Specifically, it increases the intensity with which the emotions of the people in the photos impact the emotional state of the participant. So, could MDMA help people with antisocial behavior experience emotional empathy and transform their behavior? During development, there are critical periods for the development of certain skills, such as language. Whatever happens to us during this critical early period will set the stage for the direction in which the brain will develop, and once this critical period has passed, it is difficult to change that which we have learned. In the case concerning us here, there also seems to be a critical period for learning to perceive social interactions as indifferent, rewarding, or threatening. Criminology shows how people who have committed heinous crimes have often had childhoods filled with neglect or abuse. It is unlikely that MDMA can reverse something so fundamentally established in childhood, and, to date, no studies have been carried out exploring this directly. However, a study in rats led by Romain Nardou in 2019 offers some intriguing results. In this study, MDMA was administered to adult rats no longer within the critical period for learning about social reward. The results showed that, despite being outside the animal's critical period, MDMA resulted in social reward-related learning equal to that obtained during the rat's critical period. Could these results suggest that the effects of MDMA promote a state in some way similar to the critical period of social learning? If so, could MDMA then activate empathy and the ability to form gratifying social bonds in people with antisocial behavior who were unable to form them during their critical period? This is a fascinating question to which we do not yet have an answer.

The increased empathy promoted by MDMA manifests itself through behavior. In particular, MDMA increases prosocial behavior, something that has also been demonstrated using laboratory tasks. During these, the participant has to decide how they will distribute, between themselves and a group of people, a prize that they will be granted at the end of the experiment. The results show that, when allocating the resources of the prize under the influence of MDMA, participants minimize the difference between that which they will receive and that which they will offer to the others. In other words, it seems as if the well-being of the group gains importance to the individual. And this makes sense. After all, in this highly empathic state, the well-being of the individual is highly impacted by the well-being of the group.

But MDMA's effects go beyond empathy and prosocial behavior. Its effects also reach oneself, giving rise, as happens under classic psychedelics, to a deep sense of self-compassion. For this reason, a few years later, David Nichols (who, by the way, has been responsible for synthesizing a large part of the MDMA used in current studies) preferred to call this type of substance an "entactogenic," in reference to its capacity to produce (*gen* in Greek) an internal (*en* "within" in Greek) touch (*tactus* in Latin).

Particularly noticeable is also the strong impact this molecule has on people's mood and emotional state. Not only does it promote feelings of supreme happiness and euphoria with an intensity similar to that of classic psychedelics, it also does so with a greater consistency than the latter. Basically, we could say that it is harder not to enjoy an MDMA trip than it is one with classic psychedelics. That said, the maximum enjoyment that can be achieved on a good psychedelic trip tends to be somewhat greater than that on MDMA, but this is not necessarily a very big difference. Undoubtedly, MDMA can generate a profound feeling of well-being.

In studying its clinical applications, we also saw how the effects of MDMA seemed to significantly decrease social anxiety. Instead, it seems to increase closeness and trust between individuals, something that has not only been demonstrated through questionnaires and interviews. Researchers have gone so far as to administer MDMA to octopuses!

The octopus is a highly antisocial animal that tends to avoid contact with other individuals of its species. However, under the effects of MDMA, they seemed to increase their search for friendly contact and closeness with each other, something that would be impossible if the octopus felt threatened. And this effect has also been corroborated in rodents.

Without knowing its precise mechanism of action, MDMA seems to be able to suppress fear, but it cannot be considered an anxiolytic as such, since, although it is not common, cases of increased anxiety or even panic attacks have indeed been reported. It must work through another anxiolytic mechanism that we have not yet deciphered. Be that as it may, this molecule seems to be able to lower the individual's defense mechanisms, though in this case, such an effect is not accompanied by the characteristic deconstruction of one's identity underpinning classic psychedelics' effects. Nevertheless, and as we shall see, MDMA can still profoundly transform people.

Neurobiology of MDMA

In what specific ways is MDMA interacting with the brain to produce its characteristic subjective effects?

Like classic psychedelics, the MDMA molecule exerts its action mainly through the serotonergic system. However, this action differs markedly from that of molecules such as psilocybin, DMT, or LSD. While, as we have seen, the latter produce a massive release of glutamate by interacting with the serotonin 2A receptor located in cortical neurons, MDMA interacts with the transporter proteins located in the membranes of both the axon terminal and the vesicles (see figure 3) of serotonergic, noradrenergic and, to a lesser extent, dopaminergic neurons. The result of such interactions is a massive release of all these neurotransmitters but, how exactly does this occur?

In figure 51, you can see how the molecular structure of MDMA shares strong similarities with that of these neurotransmitters. Because of this, after MDMA intake, this substance is capable of first interacting with the reuptake transporter proteins located in the membranes of axon terminals (i.e., the transporter proteins involved in reintroducing neurotransmitters from the synaptic cleft back to the interior of the neuron). These reuptake proteins perceive MDMA as if it were the neurotransmitter in question, and, as such, introduce it into the neuron. But once here, MDMA is only partially recognized as the neurotransmitter: it binds to the transporter proteins located in the vesicles' membranes,[1] but blocks them, precluding the entry of both the MDMA molecule and the neurotransmitters. This results in the neurotransmitters accumulating in a dispersed manner in the axon terminal.

How does the neurotransmitters' massive release into the synaptic cleft take place, given that the vesicles are not filled up with neurotransmitters? The answer is that just as when reuptake proteins in the neuronal membrane detect a high concentration of neurotransmitters in the synaptic cleft they transport them back inside the neuron, when they instead detect a high concentration of neurotransmitters inside the neuron, they transport them out to the synaptic cleft (figure 52).

The end result of this interaction between MDMA and the membranes' transporter proteins is a more uncontrolled and intense release of neurotransmitters into the synaptic cleft than that usually produced by

---

1. For more information, please refer to the section in chapter 1 on the neuroanatomy of the neuron and to figure 3.

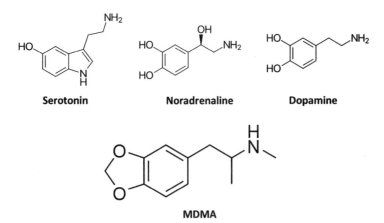

Figure 51. Molecular structure of serotonin, noradrenaline, dopamine, and MDMA.

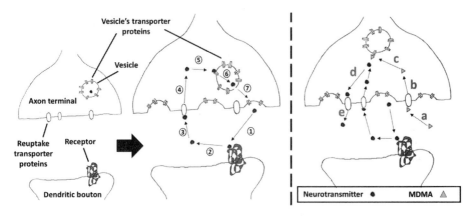

Figure 52. Effect of MDMA on the neuron. The image on the *left* shows the usual pathway a neurotransmitter follows, from the time it is expelled through the vesicle until it is reintroduced once again back into another vesicle. In the image on the *right*, step a shows MDMA anchoring itself to the reuptake-transporter receptor protein of the neuronal membrane and, step b shows how this protein transports the molecule inside the neuron. Step c shows how, once inside the neuron, this molecule is anchored to the vesicle's transporter proteins. Once anchored to these vesicular proteins, MDMA interrupts the entry of the neurotransmitter into the vesicle, causing said neurotransmitter to accumulate in a dispersed manner in the axon terminal, which in turn results in its anchoring to the intracellular part of the axon's terminal membrane reuptake proteins (step d). Finally, step e shows the neurotransmitter being transported into the synaptic cleft via the reuptake protein located in the axon's terminal membrane.

fusing the vesicles with the axon terminal. In turn, this massive release of neurotransmitters, particularly that of serotonin, triggers a series of changes that profoundly impact the limbic system and, notably, social cognition. How? By triggering the production and release of a hormone that is highly involved in the formation of social bonds: oxytocin.

There are many studies demonstrating oxytocin's strong involvement in social bond formation. A rather telling one was conducted on voles, a type of rodent. Influenced by environmental factors, this particular animal can show either a monogamous or a polygamous behavior, and studies have demonstrated that those behaving monogamously have a higher density of oxytocin receptors than those behaving polygamously. But furthermore, it turns out that when molecules that block oxytocin receptors are administered, the monogamous behavior reverts to a polygamous one! Undoubtedly, this molecule must be playing a key role in the establishment of selective and deep bonds. It is well known that this hormone is normally produced in intimate situations such as breastfeeding or sex, and also during childbirth, with the initial signals that trigger its release being originated through stimulation of the nerve endings in our skin. Such tactile stimulation specifically triggers an initial upsurge of serotonin, which in turn activates serotonin 1A receptors located in the hypothalamus. Here, it signals the production and release of oxytocin into the bloodstream. In fact, a study in rats led by Murray R. Thompson has shown that when MDMA is administered together with a molecule that blocks this serotonin receptor, there is no increase in oxytocin levels in the blood plasma and no increase in prosocial behavior in the animals either.

What exactly occurs once this hormone is released into the bloodstream and how does it influence social cognition and the formation of deep bonds?

Oxytocin can be easily administered intranasally, which has led to some very interesting and revealing studies. For example, a meta-analysis led by Rebekah Wigton in 2015 studied the results of several experiments in which neuronal activity was measured during the processing of social stimuli after the administration of this hormone and found that it had a profound impact on areas of the limbic system. For example, all studies observed a hyperactivation of the insula during the processing of social stimuli.

In addition, other PET studies, such as a study led by Arthur Lefevre in 2017, have shown how oxytocin appears to coordinate the release of serotonin in the limbic system. In this study participants were administered intranasal oxytocin together with a radioligand capable of binding to serotonin reuptake proteins (SERTs) (i.e., those located in the membranes of axon terminals). The radioligand that was employed binds to SERT with a lower affinity than serotonin so, if serotonin in the synaptic cleft increases, the amount of radioligand bound to the membrane reuptake protein should decrease, and this is precisely what the PET images show. Specifically, under the effects of oxytocin, the amount of radioligand anchored to SERT in areas of the limbic system decreased. That is, oxytocin seems to be activating serotonergic neurons in the raphe nuclei and causing them to flood areas of the limbic system with serotonin, consequently, preventing the binding of the radioligand. This effect of oxytocin over the release of serotonin is interesting, as we know that this neurotransmitter is highly involved in mood regulation and in the establishment of social hierarchies. From lobsters to primates, the release of serotonin promotes greater self-confidence. Could this be the reason why MDMA also has a positive impact on self-esteem? It seems likely that this is the case!

In addition, several studies in rats have shown how the prosocial behaviors of MDMA are reversed if the serotonin 1a receptor is blocked, possibly because, as we saw, this receptor is responsible for signaling oxytocin release in neurons of the hypothalamus. Not surprisingly, when oxytocin receptors are blocked directly, this behavior is also reversed. Perhaps oxytocin, which is usually released through intimate contact, positions the person in a state related to the safety provided by family, partners, good friends, thereby reducing stress, generating well-being, and increasing self-esteem. From this state empathy and prosocial behavior can now emerge. It is possible then that, by indirectly promoting the release of oxytocin thanks to the serotonin release, MDMA transfers animals to this safe space.

But the effect of oxytocin goes beyond its effect on the serotonergic system. Once in the bloodstream, this hormone also promotes the release of dopamine from the ventral tegmental area. In chapter 1 we saw that this area highly innervates the nucleus accumbens of the ventral striatum, as well as other parts of the limbic system, flooding them with dopamine, which is, in turn, strongly implicated in the reward system and thus, in pleasure and addiction. But what role does dopamine play in the context of social cognition? In this particular case, this neurotransmitter appears to be involved in the processing of social reward. That is, it is responsible for generating attachment and desire for proximity. In fact, some studies investigating romantic love have found a strong activation of this dopaminergic area when participants who consider themselves to be in love look at pictures of their respective partners. Now you can understand why attachment or social networking may behave like an addiction. It's an addiction to social stimuli!

In summary, MDMA appears to be activating systems involved in social cognition, positively impacting interpersonal relationships.

MDMA's Psychotherapeutic Properties

Research exploring the success of different psychotherapeutic methods shows that the best predictor of psychotherapy's success is not the method employed, but the quality of the therapeutic alliance formed between therapist and patient. Thus, MDMA's effects on deep bond formation and relaxation of defense mechanisms might allow it to accelerate psychotherapeutic processes in a rather general way. More specifically, the molecule's characteristics make it a fantastic candidate for treating social anxiety, interpersonal conflict resolution, and posttraumatic stress disorder. Let's see why.

Social Anxiety

Oxytocin and dopamine strongly underpin the formation of deep and selective social bonds and the formation of such bonds is highly related to fear: we could never form a deep and authentic bond with a person by whom we felt threatened! Feeling safe is, of course, a prerequisite and, although the precise way in which this occurs is still uncertain, we know that amygdala activity is primarily regulated by serotonergic projections. We can begin to sense why MDMA may have a strong therapeutic impact on social anxiety. Under the effects of this molecule, other people cease to be perceived as threatening, perhaps because, on the one hand, it increases self-confidence, and, on the other, promotes the release of hormones such as oxytocin related to safe environments.

Conflict Resolution

Although during the psychedelic renaissance no studies have yet been conducted exploring MDMA's application in conflict resolution, prior to its prohibition, MDMA was indeed employed during couples' therapy. By producing a highly empathic, prosocial, and relaxed, yet alert, state, this molecule presents ideal properties that facilitate the emergence of authentic and honest conversations. In such a state, one truly wants to understand the other person's feelings and, setting aside the pride or resentment that usually drives defensive reactions to criticism, listens carefully. It would not be surprising if this was also useful during family therapy. And on a sad day like today, the seventh day since Vladimir Putin began invading Ukraine, one cannot help but wonder how the course of historical events would be altered if, during the negotiations, the aggressors were under the effects of MDMA. Perhaps this is naïve thinking. I don't know. But it is certainly frustrating not to be able to test it! Would they show more empathy toward the other members of the table, and if so, would such prosocial effects linger after the MDMA had washed off? Wouldn't it be extremely interesting to see their reactions?

Post-Traumatic Stress Disorder (PTSD)

Regardless of the reduction in social anxiety, the increase in empathy and the facilitation of a good therapeutic alliance, the feelings that these molecules promote seem particularly useful for post-traumatic stress disorder. Why? In what specific ways might the phenomenological and biological characteristics of MDMA be facilitating the treatment of this particular disorder?

As the name suggests, post-traumatic stress disorder emerges in the aftermath of a traumatic event. Symptoms do not appear immediately after the event but often begin within a few months. Or even a year! And when they do, they produce painful flashbacks that vividly take the individual back to the traumatic memory, causing tremendous panic. With each flashback, the experience is relived, leading to particularly high suicide rates. Theories postulate that such flashbacks occur because the traumatic event has failed to become properly integrated into the individual's memory and personal history. We could say that the hippocampus usually stores memories within a database built of separate files. While nontraumatic memories are stored within a specific file where the memory in question is orderly organized, traumatic memories are not fully integrated into their own individual file, and, instead, remain fragmented and scattered all over the place, spilling over onto other memories. The consequence of this is that, if the environment contains a stimulus that in some way, even if only subconsciously, has been associated with the traumatic event, such stimulus will be able to activate the specific fragment of the traumatic memory that contains it and trigger a flashback. This can occur at any time and no voluntary control over its appearance is possible, so, in an attempt to avoid exposure to possible triggering stimuli, it is common for people suffering from PTSD to start withdrawing from the world, which ends up causing a pronounced disability. Nightmares and intrusive thoughts related to the traumatic event also start to appear and the person begins to find themselves in a constant state of alertness. Not only do they need to protect themselves from potentially threatening stimuli from the outside world. They must also make a constant effort to try to calm the scary beast that lies within them, which results in many resorting to substance abuse. The quality of sleep also worsens and, little by little, mood deteriorates, impacting not only one's self-image but also one's social relationships. The person eventually isolates themselves from family and friends, ultimately leading to depression.

See how Amy Oestreicher, known for her motivational talks and books where she shares the way in which she overcame the disorder, expresses what it felt like to suffer from PTSD:

It becomes difficult to deal with everyday life because you've hid your soul in a dark corner so it doesn't have to face the dangerous world of the Trauma. Without your soul, you are only half a person, a machine who is constantly running from reality.

When shocking events that radically change our life story happen to us, the brain cannot process all the information at once. It needs time to fully integrate it into its reality. Think about when the pandemic started. It seemed unreal. The same thing is happening now as I write this in the face of a possible world nuclear war. I wish that by the time you read this there will be peace. May we never ever be forced to integrate the reality war victims are faced with into our daily lives and may all those affected by it find the strength to grow through their pain.

The prolonged process of integration does not only occur when the information pertaining to the extraordinary event is negative. For example, it may also occur when a new family member is born. In order to integrate the new information, your memory needs to recall from time to time the new context in which it finds itself ("I'm an aunt!"), until the information becomes integrated into the individual's personal history and no longer feels surprising or shocking. However, during negative events, the amygdala is overactivated and signals to the hypothalamus the need to generate a hormonal cocktail capable of preparing the body to either flee or fight. Among these ingredients we find glucocorticoids, and the amygdala, hippocampus, and prefrontal cortex all have abundant receptors for them. These play a key role in memory formation, as shown by studies in rats in which, by blocking these receptors via specific molecules, the learning of emotional information was hindered.

It is important for living organisms to encode well that which in the past was rewarding, and also that which was damaging and threatening. Failure to encode such information correctly could mark the difference between life and death. Hence, the important role of glucocorticoids in memory formation. However, the efficiency with which we encode new memories does not increase linearly with the concentration levels of glucocorticoids in the bloodstream. Rather, it's a matter of reaching an optimal point, meaning that, when stress levels are above or below this point, encoding efficiency is hindered. During traumatic events, large amounts of glucocorticoids are released, possibly interfering with the processing of information during the experience and its subsequent integration into memory.

It is not uncommon to experience a sudden eruption of trauma-related mnemonic fragments after traumatic events, this possibly being an attempt by the brain to integrate them. However, not everyone develops PTSD. While some people may be more predisposed to developing this disorder than others, it is believed that the way in which one deals with those early flashbacks plays an important role. As each flashback generates deep psychological pain and stress, many people choose to engage in avoidance behaviors, but this is the opposite of what one should do. In order to overcome the disorder, the reprocessing of the experience, both cognitively and emotionally, is necessary. Only in this way can the brain orderly store the event in its own differentiated file.

Cognitive-behavioral therapy, among others, is often used for this purpose. In an attempt to modify the cognitive frameworks through which the patient understands the traumatic event and integrate it into their life's story, during these sessions they must make the effort to recollect the traumatic memory and organize it in their mind. And, if during this process, the person succeeds in conveying meaning to the pain associated with the traumatic event, even exponential personal growth can occur. In fact, among all the people who suffer from this disorder, there is a group of them who manage to turn their trauma into their fortress and experience what is known as post-traumatic growth.

But not only the mind has to process the trauma. The body does too. That is, not only does the experience have to be integrated into one's narrative and declarative memory (based on the connections between the hippocampus, the limbic thalamic nuclei, and the default mode network). It also has to be integrated into somatic and emotional memory, something that possibly occurs through modifying the relationship between the amygdala, the hippocampus, and the insula. In fact, although we do not fully understand this mechanism, we know that the connectivity between the insula and the amygdala significantly predicts people's anxiety levels. The greater the connectivity, the greater the anxiety. To integrate the event emotionally and physically, somatic therapies are used to address, for example, bodily tension or physical pain. Different breathing techniques are also applied (e.g., relaxing, holotropic). The body and mind are one, and the state of the system can be modified in both directions. The mind can stress or relax the body, and the body can stress or relax the mind.

Finally, conventional psychotherapies frequently employ prolonged exposure to innocuous stimuli that, due to having been associated with the traumatic event, are nonetheless being perceived as threatening by the brain. By being re-exposed to them in a new and safe context, this therapy intends for the patient to "unlearn" that such neutral stimuli pose a threat. That is, prolonged exposure allows them to be reconsolidated into a new mnemonic space that is separated from the traumatic event.

These three therapies (cognitive, somatic, and prolonged exposure) are the most effective in treating PTSD, but it is an extremely painful and slow process, and the drop-out rate is high. In addition, it is also common for the mind to dissociate from reality in order to protect itself from the painful information, which makes healing notoriously difficult.

This is where MDMA comes in. The self-confidence and good mood that the substance produces, accompanied by the therapeutic environment, allows the person to feel safe, which, even in those who are dissociated, facilitates their coping with memories and emotions linked to the traumatic experience. In this way, information processing is achieved, significantly accelerating the integration of difficult emotions and memories, and thus the psychotherapeutic process. For example, one participant in a study led by William Barone in 2019 compared MDMA therapy with other therapies as follows:

> When I did the MDMA study it was exactly what they were trying to get me to do (in other therapies) . . . but I guess in such a slow pace . . . and then I got on the rocket ship (of) the MDMA . . . I still got a ways to go, but I definitely accelerated from where I was, no doubt.

And another patient expressed his experience during MDMA therapy as follows:

I think that the MDMA gave me the ability to feel as though I was capable and safe of tackling the issues. Whereas before I feared those thoughts and I tried to avoid them at all times, and avoid things that reminded me of those thoughts, I think it allowed me to feel safe in my space. Of being able to fight it. I felt like I had the ability and tools, whereas before I was unarmed, unarmored, and had no support. And this type of environment, with [the therapists], the catalyst drug, and everything else, it felt as though I had backup. Now it was safe and I had my tools and weapons to be able to tackle the obstacles that I never had before.

Similarly, another participant mentioned in an article from *The Science Explorer* written by Kelly Tatera said the following:

Under the influence of MDMA, I was able to talk about and work through these things without having that physiological reaction . . . It kind of rewires the brain back to baseline before the PTSD.

It is not that the euphoria makes the process pleasant. Facing the traumatic event is still painful, but, as with psychedelics, this euphoria is complemented with feelings of love for others and oneself, which make the person feel protected during this painful process.

What is it that neuroimaging studies find? When the effects of MDMA have been studied within the functional MRI scanner, all results suggest that the molecule attenuates the activation of areas involved in signaling threat and negative emotions. For example, one study on healthy participants found an attenuation of the amygdala during the processing of angry faces. What is more, it also found that, during the processing of happy faces, areas of the ventral striatum highly involved in the processing of reward showed increased activation. Could these results, therefore, be reflecting how under MDMA, positive stimuli cause greater pleasure and negative stimuli cause less psychological distress? Another study measuring the affective impact of recollecting positive and negative autobiographical memories also pointed to this direction. While under the effects of MDMA, recollecting positive memories caused more positive feelings, recollecting negative ones caused fewer negative ones. In addition, neuroimaging showed that, during the processing of negative memories, MDMA caused an attenuation of the anterior temporal lobe. This area is highly proximal and highly connected to the amygdala, and its activity was also correlated with the intensity of the negative affect experienced during recollection of the negative memories. The lower the activation, the lower the negative affect. Finally, other studies have also found a reduction in basal amygdala activity during rest, and again, levels of activity in this area were correlated with the subjective effects of the experience. Clearly, for one reason or another, though possibly through the release of serotonin, there appears to be lower activity in the areas involved in processing negative emotions under the effects of MDMA.

What about the prefrontal cortex? We have already discussed how top-down projections from the prefrontal cortex to the amygdala play a key role in regulating the activation of this subcortical structure. Does MDMA increase activity in this area? This is what neuroimaging studies seem to show! In particular, MDMA seems to increase activity in the orbital and ventromedial prefrontal cortex, areas highly connected to the amygdala and ventral striatum. Could these results indicate that MDMA facilitates emotion regulation by activating the top-down projections from the prefrontal cortex to the amygdala? That is, does MDMA make it harder for the amygdala to conduct the mental act within us? In people with post-traumatic stress disorder, there seems to be a dominance of bottom-up signals going from the amygdala to the prefrontal cortex over top-down signals going in the opposite direction (i.e., from the prefrontal cortex to the amygdala). This is reflected by hypoactivation of the prefrontal cortex and hyperactivation of the amygdala, which is characteristic of this and other anxiety-related disorders. Therefore, the effects that MDMA seems to have on the amygdala and the prefrontal cortex in healthy people could be highly beneficial in improving emotional regulation in those suffering from PTSD and, more generally, anxiety.

In addition, MDMA also appears to affect connectivity between the hippocampus and the amygdala, which tends to be lower in people with PTSD. Some have speculated that this reduced connectivity may relate to the difficulty in recontextualizing and reconsolidating that those innocuous stimuli that were present during the traumatic event are not truly threatening. That is, it may reflect the person's inability to "unlearn" the association between that stimulus and the threat posed by the traumatic event. Whether this pattern of reduced connectivity between the amygdala and the hippocampus arises as a result of the disorder or whether it may precede it and act as a predisposing factor, is unknown, but whatever the case may be, MDMA seems to increase such a connectivity pattern. Could this be reflecting the way in which MDMA activates traumatic memory reconsolidation? This would, of course, have major implications for this disorder, where a key part of the treatment resides in eliminating the pathological association between neutral stimuli and danger formed during the traumatic event.

Several animal studies also support the notion that MDMA accelerates learning and model updating. For example, when mice that have been conditioned to fear an innocuous (e.g., sound) stimuli (by always presenting it together with an aversive stimulus (e.g., electric shock), begin to be exposed to it without the presence of the aversive stimulus, MDMA administration seems to accelerate the relearning of what the neutral stimulus entails (i.e., not a threat). In other words, mice receiving MDMA stop being afraid of it more quickly than those receiving a placebo, suggesting that this molecule is facilitating the memory reconsolidation of this innocuous stimulus. Along these lines, other studies have also shown that MDMA activates the production of the neurotrophic growth factor (BDNF), key to neuroplasticity, ultimately modifying the connections between the amygdala and the hippocampus and facilitating this important emotional updating.

In short, MDMA not only facilitates the reprocessing of the traumatic experience by making exposure to the associated memories less psychologically painful. It also appears to be acting directly at a biological level, activating pathways involved in neuroplasticity in key areas linked to emotional memory.

From the theory of predictive coding, we could say that the reprocessing of traumatic memory in the safe and therapeutic environment offered by MDMA-assisted psychotherapy allows the generation of a powerful prediction error, product of the discrepancy detected between the threatening model of the world built after the trauma and the incoming safe information. In this way, the patient can truly realize that the stimuli in question are no longer threatening and update the model.

Look at how one participant expressed this process in an article written by Kelley McMillan in Marie Claire magazine:

> I felt as if I was literally reprogramming my brain and confronting all the fixed thought patterns and belief structures that were keeping the PTSD in place, that were making me relive the past over and over again. I was able to file those memories in the past.

Finally, studies have shown that patients with PTSD show decreased cognitive and emotional empathy, which, when reversed under the effects of MDMA, can provide the individual with a new platform from which to feel and communicate with others, ultimately allowing them to regain pleasure from social relationships. And while MDMA does not affect the semantic network and does not result in the deconstruction of meanings and identity, the new emotional perspective that it provides can facilitate moments of insight that promote lasting change and transform the way in which the individual perceives themselves.

Overall, the phenomenology of MDMA mirrors states associated with moments of intimacy and security. In this way, the molecule is able to offer the individual a profound state of well-being in which empathy and trust are increased, not only in oneself, but also in others. This allows the ego's defense mechanisms to be reduced, thus enhancing the therapeutic alliance and interpersonal relationships.

In the specific case of post-traumatic stress, inducing this safe state of mind during the therapeutic process offers the person the opportunity to finally be able to process the traumatic experience in depth and integrate it into their life story. This allows them to reconsolidate the memory in a new place within their psyche. A place where neutral stimuli, previously capable of triggering painful flashbacks, are no longer perceived as threatening. A re-learning takes place based on unlearning those associations that were recorded in the memory during the traumatic event but are no longer relevant. In this way, MDMA-assisted therapy allows the individual to regain his or her life and become the person they were before the traumatic event.

References for Further Study

Barone W, Beck J, Mitsunaga-Whitten M, Perl P. 2019. Perceived benefits of MDMA-assisted psychotherapy beyond symptom reduction: qualitative follow-up study of a clinical trial for individuals with treatment-resistant PTSD. Journal of Psychoactive Drugs 51(2):199–208.

Bedi G, Phan KL, Angstadt M, De Wit H. 2009. Effects of MDMA on sociability and neural response to social threat and social reward. Psychopharmacology 207(1):73–83.

Carhart-Harris RL, Wall MB, Erritzoe D, Kaelen M, Ferguson B, De Meer I, Tanner M, Bloomfield M, Williams TM, Bolstridge M, et al. 2014. The effect of acutely administered MDMA on subjective and BOLD-fMRI responses to favourite and worst autobiographical memories. International Journal of Neuropsychopharmacology 17(4):527–540.

Dahlgren MK, Laifer LM, VanElzakker MB, Offringa R, Hughes KC, Staples-Bradley LK, Dubois SJ, Lasko NB, Hinojosa CA, Orr SP, et al. 2018. Diminished medial prefrontal cortex activation during the recollection of stressful events is an acquired characteristic of PTSD. Psychological Medicine 48(7):1128–1138.

Edsinger E, Dölen G. 2018. A conserved role for serotonergic neurotransmission in mediating social behavior in octopus. Current Biology 28(19): 3136–3142.

Francati V, Vermetten E, Bremner JD. 2007. Functional neuroimaging studies in posttraumatic stress disorder: review of current methods and findings. Depression and Anxiety 24(3):202–218.

Gamma A, Buck A, Berthold T, Hell D, Vollenweider FX. 2000. 3,4-methylenedioxymethamphetamine (MDMA) modulates cortical and limbic brain activity as measured by [H215O]-PET in healthy humans. Neuropsychopharmacology 23(4):388–395.

Holze F, Vizeli P, Müller F, Ley L, Duerig R, Varghese N, Eckert A, Borgwardt S, Liechti ME. 2020. Distinct acute effects of LSD, MDMA, and D-amphetamine in healthy subjects. Neuropsychopharmacology 45(3):462–471.

Hysek CM, Schmid Y, Simmler LD, Domes G, Heinrichs M, Eisenegger C, Preller KH, Quednow BB, Liechti ME. 2014. MDMA enhances emotional empathy and prosocial behavior. Social Cognitive and Affective Neuroscience 9(11):1645–1652.

Kamilar-Britt P, Bedi G. 2015. The prosocial effects of 3, 4-methylenedioxymethamphetamine (MDMA): controlled studies in humans and laboratory animals. Neuroscience & Biobehavioral Reviews 57:433–446.

Kuypers KP, Dolder PC, Ramaekers JG, Liechti ME. 2017. Multifaceted empathy of healthy volunteers after single doses of MDMA: a pooled sample of placebo-controlled studies. Journal of Psychopharmacology 31(5):589–598.

Lefevre A, Richard N, Jazayeri M, Beuriat PA, Fieux S, Zimmer L, Duhamel J-R, Sirigu A. 2017. Oxytocin and serotonin brain mechanisms in the non-human primate. Journal of Neuroscience 37(28):6741–6750.

McMillan K. 2015. Is Ecstasy the Key to Treating Women with PTSD? Marie Claire (available online).

Nardou R, Lewis EM, Rothhaas R, Xu R, Yang A, Boyden E, Dölen G. 2019. Oxytocin-dependent reopening of a social reward learning critical period with MDMA. Nature 569(7754):116–120.

Stein DJ, Vythilingum B. 2009. Love and attachment: the psychobiology of social bonding. CNS Spectrums 14(5):239–242.

Thompson MR, Li KM, Clemens KJ, Gurtman CG, Hunt GE, Cornish JL, McGregor IS. 2004. Chronic fluoxetine treatment partly attenuates the long-term anxiety and depressive symptoms induced by MDMA ('Ecstasy') in rats. Neuropsychopharmacology 29(4):694–704.

Tatera K. 2016. Meet a Former Soldier Who Overcame His Life-Threatening PTSD With MDMA-Therapy. The Science Explorer. Can be accessed on the internet.

Thompson MR, Hunt GE, McGregor IS. 2009. Neural correlates of MDMA ("Ecstasy")-induced social interaction in rats. Social Neuroscience 4(1):60–72.

Wigton R, Radua J, Allen P, Averbeck B, Meyer-Lindenberg A, McGuire P, Shergill SS, Fusar-Poli P. 2015. Neurophysiological effects of acute oxytocin administration: systematic review and meta-analysis of placebo-controlled imaging studies. Journal of Psychiatry and Neuroscience 40(1):E1–E22.

Young KA, Liu Y, Wang Z. 2008. The neurobiology of social attachment: a comparative approach to behavioral, neuroanatomical, and neurochemical studies. Comparative Biochemistry and Physiology Part C: Toxicology & Pharmacology 148(4):401–410.

6

The Future of Psychedelia

I will never forget the first time I experienced the lysergic magic. It was September 2012 at a festive adventure in the mountains of Córdoba, Spain, accompanied by my dear friends and huge characters, Budy and Lape, who brought with them a beautiful person, Angie. And Goku. There is no dog with more personality, elegance, and gentleness!

I learned many things on that trip. I learned that another way of being in the present moment was possible, and that the human experience goes beyond the frenetic, rational, and purely mental level in which, I suddenly discovered, I had been trapped all this time. I also learned that I need not be looking for answers and solving problems at all times. That the most important thing was to know how to laugh at this cosmic joke called life. And to be thankful. To "embody gratitude" through the conscious participation with the existential whole that we are all woven into. Through perceiving the unfolding of the exquisite *psytrance* music that flooded the experience like an intriguing tale, I also learned how to dance. And I learned that by paying attention to the sensations of our breathing we can soothe the spirit. Later, I realized that I had connected with Buddhist teachings related to being present: nonseparation, acceptance, nonjudgment, and gratitude.

Without ever paying any attention to it or even perceiving it as a problem, I have always been a rather restless person. I couldn't even begin to fathom that such levels of inner calm and serenity as those experienced for at least the two weeks following this trip were possible. I felt an unbelievable peace of mind! And now that my usual hyper-activity was no longer burning up all of my seemingly endless internal energy, an astonishing vitality ensued. Not an inch of fear existed within me either. I was invincible.

I won't lie. Accepting that my "afterglow" was fading away was not easy. I had thought it would last forever! I guess some people can get a little lost during this phase, in the struggle against the return to the old state of mind. It was a struggle to recover the peace acquired after the trip, and the disappointment and frustration felt at every failed attempt to recover it, led to ultimately forgetting the most important lessons of all: to flow, not to judge, and to be grateful.

How could such an exquisite and enriching experience as the one I had just had be illegal? It didn't make sense! Such incongruence unleashed alarm bells inside me—a distrust toward the authorities who had banned and stigmatized it. "These substances could transform humanity, they must want us numbed and enslaved," I would think. It would not be surprising if this reasoning explained the high number of psychedelic users that believe in conspiracy theories. After all, why would one continue trusting authorities who had gone to such lengths to stigmatize substances capable of generating such spiritual well-being? And many of us have joked about carrying out psychedelic terrorism:

"Let's lace the water in parliament with LSD and MDMA! That way the politicians will do acts of kindness!" "And the water of the whole city! Everyone should have this experience, at least once in their lifetime! They must wake up and learn that another way of being is possible!"

This "psychedelic fever" is not uncommon and perfectly under-standable. Imagine, all of a sudden, feeling a profound understanding of the teachings contained within an ancient philosophy you had never before paid attention to! Or no longer being afraid to look at people in the eyes and communicate from your heart! No wonder you wish the same for all humankind and in blissful ignorance, begin making an uncontrolled apology for consumption of these substances. However, with time one learns that the integration of these tools into society is not a simple matter and that caution must be taken.

A Warning on Set, Setting, and the Wake

The state to which these substances transport us facilitates a series of beneficial events that can promote wisdom, but whether or not such potential manifests itself depends on many variables. Set and setting, the popular psychedelic terminology that refers to how the internal and external factors influence the psychedelic experience, are key. Set and setting, and let me add, the wake.

The positive therapeutic outcomes we have studied throughout the book don't depend solely on the substance, nor do they depend solely on whether one feels safe in the environment (*setting*) in which it is being consumed—something we have already insisted on. It also depends on the individual characteristics of the person and on how one deals with the death of the ego when such a death begins to lurk. Will you surrender to the experience and freely navigate the stream that the substance wants to take you on, or will you resist and divert it from its path? What attitude and intention are you bringing to the journey? What is your mind*set?*

These issues of *set* and *setting* will make a big difference in determining the quality of the experience. This is why (even in a controlled environment) such an experience may not necessarily be beneficial for everyone. For example, someone who is overly controlling may experience a constant inner battle as they find themselves unable to surrender to the experience and let go. Previous psychological preparation before embarking on such an altered state is essential.

It is also essential to be well informed about the effects that these molecules might cause. I have personally known of several people who have had a bad trip on psilocybin or LSD because they were unaware of the ego-dissolution phenomenon. For good reason it has been called "the death of the ego" because this is precisely how it is perceived: as a death. If someone is unaware of this quality of the experience, when such a sensation appears, it may be interpreted as a physical death, unleashing a deep anguish in the person as they perceive the unbearable suffering that their death will cause to their loved ones!

And now, the wake. The psychedelic experience can present us with some fantastic tools, such as our capability of existing in a different state of mind, but how much we strive to apply those tools on a daily basis is what will largely determine its long-term benefits. The nurturing of a calm and mindful presence must be carefully and patiently trained. Hence, this is why daily meditative practices can be very helpful, since they can, in a nonchaotic and orderly way, help us remember to exercise the capacity we have, if only for a few seconds, to stop, feel, and connect with the present moment. Finally, it is crucial that as these substances reach the mainstream, we do not communicate a message to the masses that leads to unrealistic expectations. Psychotherapists are already seeing how expectations of this kind can pose a dangerous problem for people who perceive these molecules as being their last hope. If such expectations are not fulfilled (and remember, these molecules don't necessarily deliver what one hopes), suicidal ideation or suicidal behavior may increase. Furthermore, by trying to steer the experience in a predetermined direction, high expectations (or expectations of any kind) can also generate a resistance that derails one from the substance's natural path. It is essential to let the substance guide you, and you must also know that, when the environment, attitude, or prior preparation are not adequate, the intensity reached in these states of consciousness can be detrimental to the stability of the psyche, especially with classic psychedelics.

In this sense, and despite its use nowadays being more heavily prosecuted than that of classic psychedelics, MDMA is a safer substance. However, MDMA does have a higher potential for abuse. Even though in therapeutic contexts, and more specifically during post-traumatic stress disorder therapy, the MDMA experience is not necessarily easy or pleasant, MDMA's effects are much easier to navigate than those of classic psychedelics, which makes it a rather "appetizing" and tempting substance within recreational settings. Moreover, while studies exploring the neurotoxic potential of MDMA have produced ambiguous results, it is likely that while it is psychologically safer than classic psychedelics (which do not appear to produce physical damage to nervous tissue and with which it is virtually impossible to overdose on), the same is not true when it comes to physical damage.

Although MDMA overdoses are extremely rare, its physiological effects, combined with the hot and dance-like environment in which it is often consumed, can pose a serious health risk. Due to the consumers' ignorance regarding such risks, this molecule has led to the deaths of more people than it should have. In addition to having potentially life-threatening cardiovascular effects, MDMA interferes with body temperature regulation on the one hand and causes fluid retention on the other. Such water retention combined with the physical exertion of dancing makes us feel dehydrated, which leads us to drink plenty of water; but when dancing and sweating, the body not only eliminates water, it also exudes salts. Due to the physiological effects of MDMA, the water we ingest will not be excreted at the same rate as that of the salts, leading to an ion imbalance of potentially deadly consequences. For this reason, not plain water but fluids containing electrolytes, such as isotonic drinks, should be drunk when consuming MDMA in a hot and physically active environment. After all, it is not necessarily the substance that kills, but the ignorance surrounding its safe use, which is largely a product of prohibition. That said, some studies also suggest that excessive consumption of MDMA may cause damage to nerve tissue and impairment of cognitive functions, such as memory, so particular care should be taken not to abuse this ecstatic molecule.

Future Clinical Applications

Having reviewed the phenomenology and neurobiology of these substances, as well as their dangers and benefits, several questions arise: Could they also help in the treatment of other psychopathologies that have so far been excluded from studies? Should this type of therapy be the patient's last medical option or, if psychologically prepared and willing, should it, instead, be one of the first? After all, these substances seem to produce fewer side effects and quicker results. And, if they ultimately prove to be safe, what would their optimal place in society be? Should their use be legalized for the general public?

We have already discussed how MDMA's ability to strengthen social bonds, together with its psychologically safe profile, could make it a great tool for strengthening the therapeutic alliance and, in a rather general way, accelerate psychotherapeutic processes. But what about classic psychedelics? In which other psychopathologies, apart from those studied so far, could the powerful ego dissolution they promote be useful? In which could they be dangerous? Could they help in the treatment of anorexia nervosa, bipolar disorder, or borderline personality disorder? And in narcissistic or psychotic disorders?

To the best of my knowledge, only one additional disorder is currently undergoing clinical trials in addition to those studied so far; namely, two clinical trials are currently being conducted by the Johns Hopkins University group and by the Imperial College London group on people with anorexia nervosa. It is possible that in these people, the psychedelic experience may promote a reconnection to their body, as well as help them get to the root of their insecurity. However, these patients are characteristically highly perfectionist and have a very controlling personality. As Sandeep M. Nayak from Johns Hopkins University told me in Berlin, there is a high risk that they will find it difficult to surrender to the experience, which would prevent them from getting the maximum therapeutic benefit from it. We will have to wait and see what the results of these studies show.

What about bipolar disorder, in which the person fluctuates between depressive and euphoric states? Because the psychedelic experience can, in some cases, promote manic states, it has been considered that a high risk of switching from a depressive to a manic state exists in these patients, and as a result this disorder has been an exclusion criterion in all clinical studies so far. However, Benjamin Mudge, an expert on this disorder, which he himself suffers from, says that while the psychedelic experience may indeed worsen manic symptoms in some cases, the possibility of learning how to cope better with them through this experience also exists. In a *Psychedelics Today* podcast he shares how some of his experiences have helped him develop an awareness that allows him to detect in advance, and thus be able to curb, the onset of manic symptoms.

Perhaps a psychedelic-assisted therapy designed specifically for the depressive phase of this disorder can help people exit this state without sending them into the manic phase. Perhaps it could help them overcome their characteristic emotion-regulation disfunction.

Benjamin Mudge is currently doing his Ph.D. at Flinders University in Adelaide, South Australia, where he is, among other things, developing a specific protocol for this population. It remains to be seen what the data from a clinical trial would show. On the other hand, it is also worth mentioning that Nayak's team in 2021 has reported a possible harmful interaction between lithium, a common treatment for this psychopathology, and psychedelics. Specifically, through analyzing users' experience reports from various websites, this team detected an increase in the number of seizures in people taking psychedelics when medicated with lithium. We must be extremely cautious!

As for personality disorders, these are highly complex, and multiple types have been described. Type B personality disorders, such as borderline personality disorder or narcissistic disorder, are characterized by severe problems with emotional regulation, impulse control, and socialization, and can often be linked to traumatic experiences during childhood or adolescence. Could the psychedelic experience, therefore, be beneficial for these people? Although no clinical studies have yet been conducted, an observational study led by Elisabet Domínguez-Clavé was published in 2019 suggesting that this may be the case for those specifically suffering from borderline personality disorder. In this study, people attending an ayahuasca retreat (forty-five in total) completed several questionnaires, and the results showed that those participants who, without having borderline personality disorder, did score high on traits associated with it, achieved a significant improvement in emotional regulation scores. Perhaps the psychedelic experience could also be beneficial in treating borderline personality disorder; it just might be a matter of finding a suitable protocol.

A recurring problem in people who suffer from borderline personality disorders is their difficulty in trusting others, something that could easily trigger a state of paranoia during the altered state of consciousness. Given that these people struggle to form a good therapeutic alliance, and given that during psychedelic sessions the therapy is mainly exercised by the substance, the inner healing intelligence, and the music, could they perhaps benefit more from a "solo" psychedelic experience in which the potentially threatening presence of others is absent? Should they be left alone during the altered state of consciousness, if they so wished, and only be accompanied during the preparation and integration sessions? As we try to find the optimal approach to the use of psychedelics, we might stumble across a no-size-fits-all effect, whereby the use of these substances might be rather versatile.

As for narcissistic personality disorder, despite the fact that the psychedelic experience loosens the ego, there are cases in which, paradoxically, the ego becomes reinforced after the trip. It is not uncommon, for example, for these experiences to promote a spiritual narcissism characterized by feelings of "having been chosen" to "wake others up." When this happens, the person begins to believe that they are above those who have not yet perceived the higher truth and remain "asleep" in a "low vibrational" or "low consciousness" state. In people with narcissistic personality disorder or tendencies toward it, a mystical experience could worsen this annoying trait. Could it also promote ego inflation in those without previous narcissistic tendencies? I don't think we know for sure, but it is worth noting that experienced psychonauts such as Stanislav Grof have referred to psychedelics as non-specific amplifiers, meaning that they will amplify that which is already within oneself. Either way, beware of spiritual narcissism, both within yourself, and in the fake gurus you might stumble across!

Psychedelics are actively discouraged when it comes to psychotic disorders, as psychotic breaks following a psychedelic experience have been reported. Although they do not occur frequently and are possibly accentuated by excessive use or by use in chaotic environments, this is undoubtedly one of the greatest potential risks of these experiences. Moreover, when family trees are studied, an important genetic factor underlying psychotic disorders has been detected. We cannot rule out that for people that are genetically predisposed, the psychedelic experience may have a high risk of triggering a psychotic outbreak even with mild and controlled use. For this reason, having had a psychotic episode in the past has always been an exclusion criterion in clinical studies using psychedelics, and in some cases, even having the disorder present within one's family history is enough to be excluded.

We know that a psychotic break with reality often occurs at times of intense and prolonged stress. Could the psychedelic experience, due to its pronounced intensity, act as a stressor, tipping these people into a psychotic state for which they are genetically predisposed?

In presenting his theory of the entropic brain, Carhart-Harris has suggested that different states of consciousness can be situated along a gradient spanning from order to chaos and that while psychotic states are situated toward the "chaotic" end, other states (such as depression, addiction, anxiety, or obsession) in which the individual is stuck on a particular issue, are situated at the "order" end of the gradient. We have already seen how, by increasing entropy, psychedelics push the brain toward the chaotic end of the gradient, so it is possible that, while for patients with a tendency toward states at the orderly end of the gradient, this experience may be beneficial, it may instead be detrimental for those who naturally tend toward the chaotic end. A schematic representation of this can be seen in figure 53 or color plate 24.

In short, there are many questions we don't yet have the answers to, and much more research lies ahead, but it is possible that the effects these molecules have on the state of consciousness may improve mental health in some mental disorders and worsen it in others. I'm sure I'm not the only one impatiently waiting for more studies to expand this fascinating and potentially transformative line of research!

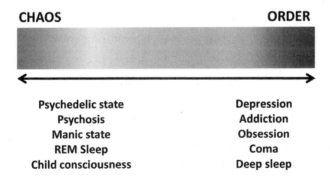

Figure 53. The gradient between chaos and order in which the state of consciousness can be situated. Image modified from the article *The Entropic Brain* by Carhart-Harris et al., published in *Frontiers in Human Neuroscience* in 2014. (See also color plate 24.)

Integration into Western Society

While in shamanic cultures the use of psychoactive substances follows a long tradition, in the West it emerged circumstantially after the accidental discovery of LSD and has developed mainly on the fringes of society, for example, at *psytrance* festivals. In light of new research, it is time to destigmatize their use and integrate them into society. But how? The optimal way to do this has yet to be discovered, but some ways can already be depicted.

It is possible that, in a society such as ours, medicalization is the most realistic and therefore the most effective way to change the status quo and end the stigmatization associated with consumption. However, many voices are critical of this approach and question whether those with a materialistic worldview are the best placed to deal with these altered states of consciousness. After all, the psychedelic experience, especially that promoted by classical psychedelics, has a weird and significant metaphysical component. Rather weird is, for example, its telepathic quality. In this state, it seems as if the people around you can, at every moment, feel everything you feel. Your fears and judgments or your joy and love. It feels as if they can, ultimately, feel your energy.[1] Could this, in part, be due to the state of heightened empathy and the feeling of connectedness to the "whole" in which we find ourselves during this state of consciousness? I don't know, but the perceived telepathic experiences certainly seem something otherworldly for which we have no explanation. In this chaotic state, it can also seem as if our consciousness has a greater capacity than we usually endow it with, to modify the material world, or at least to direct its perception. The world becomes a magical place where it's no longer only a matter of "seeing is believing" but also a matter of "believing is seeing." Because of its highly irrational and magical component, this experience has been compared to psychotic states. In fact, in the early days of research, psychiatrists consumed these substances in an attempt to better understand the delusional state of their psychotic

---

1. I think that, in a way, perceiving that our negative energies are visible to all, makes us try harder to cleanse ourselves internally. This telepathic component can also be highly stressful if we are in the presence of someone we do not trust.

patients. And, of course, in perceiving that there is something greater than oneself to which to bow with humbleness and gratitude, a spiritual component also emerges.

Given such an important metaphysical-magical-spiritual quality, are those with a biomedical approach the best suited to accompany individuals during psychedelic experiences? I personally believe that as long as the companion does not impose their worldview on the person, and as long as this does not interfere with the quality of the therapeutic alliance, this should not be a problem. After all, the therapist's function is not to ponder the ontology[2] and veracity of the experience. The therapist's function is only to reflect upon what the content of the experience might mean to the individual.

Critics of medicalization also fear that medicalization will not only be the first step toward integrating these substances into Western society but that it will also be the last, meaning that people's right to explore their consciousness will be restricted by medical institutions and regulatory agencies. In my opinion, we must, of course, not allow this to happen, but I do not believe this will be the case. Once proved that the benefits of consuming these substances outweigh the risks, there will hopefully be no justification for banning them.

Assistance by mental health professionals may be essential for people who are trapped in deep psychological distress, but how regulated should the companionship of people who do not present a severe pathology be? Should only health professionals be authorized in these cases too? And in cases where the person only wishes to work on some aspects of their personal growth or simply connect with Nature?

Several organizations such as MAPS are developing training courses for people who are professionally involved in accompanying others in their suffering and wish to work with the pharmacologically altered states caused by these substances. Although these courses are mainly aimed at psychologists and psychiatrists, people from the spiritual realm such as members of the clergy or chaplains are also being accepted. Unfortunately, at present, the prices of these courses are not easily

---

2. Ontology refers to the study of the nature of things.

affordable and extensive training is also required. While I believe that extensive training is necessary to treat people with severe psychopathologies, I don't think this is necessarily the case in other situations.

A multitude of anecdotes, as well as some scientific evidence, suggests that these experiences can be beneficial even without a formal therapist. For example, some population studies suggest that lifetime use of psychedelics is associated with less suicidal ideation, and anecdotes also exist of people with depressive tendencies who, to keep their depression at bay, embark on a psychedelic trip once every three months on their own. Perhaps psychedelics taken prophylactically could prevent people from requiring intensive psychotherapeutic support in the future. Moreover, some people cannot afford or do not want to go to therapy. Is the total absence of the psychedelic experience a better option than having it in another preferred environment freely chosen by the individual? Should the way these substances are used be limited to strictly defined protocols? Is a therapist necessarily a better companion than a good friend or a close family member? There are people who believe that, in the case of classic psychedelics, few companions are better than a cat!

Another debated question is whether training as a psychedelic therapist or psychedelic assistant should require first-person experience of these strange metaphysical realities. Perhaps this would be ideal since, by increasing their understanding of what the psychonaut is experiencing, a deeper connection between both is likely to occur. But who knows? Perhaps, having certain therapeutic skills such as being nonjudgmental and an attentive and empathetic listener suffices.

Finally, integration circles, where people can come together to share their psychedelic experiences with others, could also be a useful tool. According to Rosalind Watts, these circles are working very well and some programs, such as Beyond Experience or Footsteps, dedicated to offering retreats where participants can, in community, integrate their psychedelic experiences are already popping up.

Like any powerful tool, these molecules require a proper and responsible use, but perhaps the only requirements for consuming them should be to have certain psychological preparation, a conscious intention, and respect toward the substance.

If these substances prove to be beneficial in treating severe symptomatology in patients, why shouldn't they also facilitate personal growth in the general public? We all suffer to some degree and can improve aspects of our behavior, don't you think? And given that these substances seem to have prosocial enhancing properties, I dare to wonder whether those capable of good emotion regulation and impulse control should have to limit their use to individual and therapeutic contexts focused on one's problems. Couldn't these substances' properties instead also act as a good social adhesive used in moments of celebration? After all, what are celebrations if not ways of connecting with the community? Moreover, the intensity of these experiences can be easily manipulated through dosage, making them highly versatile.

Perhaps we should rather be striving to inform society about how to reduce the potential harms of drug intake, as organizations such as Energy Control do, and let those adults who have proven to be responsible experiment freely with their consciousness. In the hyperregulated world in which we find ourselves, I doubt that the use of these substances would be an exception. But could, for example, consumer licenses be created? And hotels that offer a safe place where support would be available if needed for those who wish to explore with altered states of consciousness?

We should be careful not to fall prey to extreme and rigid regulations that unnecessarily hinder the supply of supporting companions for those who want to feel safe while exploring their consciousness during a psychedelic trip.

To protect society from charlatans and false shamans it will, of course, be important to ensure that only capable individuals are offering these services. Even though it is difficult to predict the way in which this will become institutionalized, the psychedelic community has already developed useful tools to address some of the issues associated with the supervised use of psychedelics. For example, several websites[3] where one can leave a review of their experiences with different guides already exist.

Finally, some critics warn that these substances could become tools of control used by the state to appease society in the face of its

---

3. For example, AyaAdvisors – Ayahuasca Retreat Reviews.

enslavement; to give them a false pharmacological happiness and sense of unity, as does the "soma" described by Aldous Huxley in his dystopian novel *Brave New World*. Could this be the case? Could these substances be used to create a conformist citizenry? Personally, I don't think so. The teachings they provide us with, last beyond their pharmacological effect and are often accompanied by a motivation to change one's behavior and confront one's fears. It is not just an anxiolytic pharmacological effect like conventional antidepressants or benzodiazepines, which are already being consumed by a worrying percentage of individuals in Western society. Rather, I believe that through the inherent learning endowed within these experiences, MDMA and, above all, classic psychedelics, could charge citizens with the necessary vitality to improve the society they live in.

The problems our species faces are not few, nor do they have simple and straightforward solutions. Conflicts of interest will always be present, and selfishness, envy, greed, fear, and so forth, are all an intrinsic part of human nature. Moreover, it is often the case that the measures applied to solve a particular problem carry unforeseen consequences that create new problems impossible to predict. We should not expect these substances to be a panacea, but change is the only true constant in the universe. This is the only way we move forward. Which direction do we want to go in then? Don't you think this avenue is worth exploring?

The decisions that regulatory agencies make in the coming years will be key, not only in determining the future of psychiatry and psychotherapy. I believe that through the transformative potential that these molecules have, such decisions could also be key to transforming the whole of society, by transforming the individuals within it, little by little. Let's hope that we are allowed to explore this possibility and that we don't mess up too much along the way!

References for Further Study

Breeksema JJ, van Elk M. 2021. Working with weirdness: a response to "Moving Past Mysticism in Psychedelic Science." ACS Pharmacology & Translational Science 4(4):1471–1474.

Budisavljevic MN, Stewart L, Sahn SA, Ploth DW. 2003. Hyponatremia associated with 3, 4-methylenedioxymethylamphetamine ("Ecstasy") abuse. The American Journal of the Medical Sciences 326(2):89–93.

Burgess C, O'Donohoe A, Gill M. 2000. Agony and ecstasy: a review of MDMA effects and toxicity. European Psychiatry 15(5):287–294.

Carhart-Harris R. 2013. Psychedelic drugs, magical thinking and psychosis. Journal of Neurology, Neurosurgery and Psychiatry 84(9):e1.

Domínguez-Clavé E, Soler J, Pascual JC, Elices M, Franquesa A, Valle M, Alvarez A, Riba J. 2019. Ayahuasca improves emotion dysregulation in a community sample and in individuals with borderline-like traits. Psychopharmacology 236(2):573–580.

Nayak SM, Gukasyan N, Barrett FS, Erowid E, Griffiths RR. 2021. Classic psychedelic coadministration with lithium, but not lamotrigine, is associated with seizures: an analysis of online psychedelic experience reports. Pharmacopsychiatry 54(05):240–245.

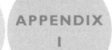

The Legal Status of Psychedelic Drugs around the World

Francisco Azorín Ortega is a lawyer specializing in legislation and jurisprudence on drugs. The information in this appendix is as up-to-date as possible as of this writing. This information is subject to change.

I. Introduction

In order to talk about legislation and jurisprudence on psychedelic drugs, the first thing we have to do is define the latter concept. Although depending on how broadly the term is interpreted it may have different meanings, on this occasion we will use a fairly broad definition of the term. Such definition will include all those substances such as LSD, DMT, psilocybin, mescaline, and 2C-B that have perceptible effects on consciousness through, noticeably, acting on the serotonin 2A neuroreceptors, as well as other substances with more dissociative psychedelic effects, such as ketamine, which acts mainly on NMDA glutamate neuroreceptors. There are also other substances classified as empathogenic-entactogenic, such as MDMA ("ecstasy"), with indirect interaction on serotonin 2A neuroreceptors, which many consider to be only semipsychedelic, but which in high doses can cause considerable psychedelic effects, like those caused by its sister substance, MDA[1], or 2C-B.

It should also be noted that these psychedelic drugs can occur as isolated molecules (either extracted or synthesized), or as part of a plant or fungus (ayahuasca, psilocybe mushrooms, cacti, and the like), or even in some animals, such as the toad *Bufo alvarius* from the Sonoran Desert (Mexico), whose glands contain the most potent of the known psychedelics, 5-MeO-DMT. Although these toads were only recently discovered to contain this molecule, 5-MeO-DMT had already been synthesized in 1936 and isolated in 1959 from the seeds of the South American tree *Anadenanthera colubrina*. Another drug that is also found in animals is DMT. On top of being present in many plants, this molecule is also found in small amounts in humans and other mammals. It, therefore, seems that these compounds may be far more important to the workings of nature than we could ever have imagined.

Today, the Western world has far more psychedelics at its disposal than could have been available in the psychedelic boom era of the 1960s and 1970s, as well as in the "Second Summer of Love," which took place in Ibiza in 1987 and was exported to the United Kingdom between 1988 and 1989 with the emergence of the semipsychedelic MDMA and "rave culture."

The explosion of the phenomenon of new designer drugs, new psychoactive substances (NPS), and their sale on the internet, as well as the growing interest in shamanic cultures and their practice in Western territories, make it necessary to review and clarify the legislation and jurisprudence that tries to deal with this social reality. The presence of a certain sector of the population that uses these substances on an occasional or recurrent basis to navigate their consciousness, reconcile and accept their traumas, free themselves from their blockages, relieve their stress or depression, and, in short, try to live in this increasingly confrontational society more consciously and peacefully is becoming increasingly evident in our current culture.

---

1. It was known in the popular slang of Spain in the 1980s and 1990s as "mescalinas" or "meskas" because of the similarity between its structure and some of its effects to those of mescaline, found in the San Pedro cactus and Mexican peyote.

The legal regime for psychedelic drugs around the world is a complex subject that has always been given to controversy and disparate interpretations, as well as constant legislative changes. In this appendix, I will attempt to provide as comprehensive and up-to-date a review as possible.

1.1 Why Were Certain Psychoactive Substances Banned?

The idea of banning all "recreational" use of certain psychoactive substances was driven by the growing influence of Anglo-American Christian Puritanism and the temperance movement against alcohol in the late 19th and early 20th centuries, which in the United States also led to the prohibition of alcohol between 1920 and 1933. The campaign for prohibition was also fuelled by racist sentiments towards immigrants from China and Mexico, who used opium and cannabis.[2]

In the 1960s, specifically in 1961, most countries in the world signed the Single Convention on Narcotic Drugs in New York, which banned opium, cannabis, and coca leaf, as well as their active ingredients and some derivatives (cocaine, morphine, and heroin). Later, new trends in the use of psychoactive drugs would emerge, such as the popularization of psychedelic substances, given that, in parallel to the promising clinical research with substances like LSD, psilocybin, and mescaline, some university professors such as Timothy Leary, writers such as Ken Kesey, and actors such as Cary Grant made their use fashionable in North America. This meant that the use of this category of substances quickly spread to the rest of the Western world, also playing an important role in the development of modern neuroscience.

With the upsurge of the nonclinical use of LSD, DMT, and psilocybin in the 1960s, associated with the hippie movement, the counterculture, and opposition to the Vietnam War, as well as their use in relation to some events reported in a very sensationalist way by the

2. Arbour, et al. 2019. Classification of psychoactive substances. Geneva (Switzerland): Global Commission on Drug Policy. Report 2019. Retrieved from the Global Commission on Drug Policy website.

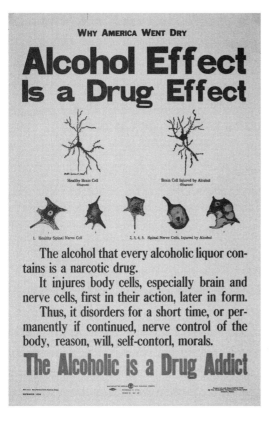

WHY AMERICA WENT DRY

Alcohol Effect
Is a Drug Effect

Healthy Brain Cell
(Diagram)

Brain Cell Injured by Alcohol
(Diagram)

1. Healthy Spinal Nerve Cell

2, 3, 4, 5. Spinal Nerve Cells, Injured by Alcohol

The alcohol that every alcoholic liquor contains is a narcotic drug.

It injures body cells, especially brain and nerve cells, first in their action, later in form.

Thus, it disorders for a short time, or permanently if continued, nerve control of the body, reason, will, self-contorl, morals.

The Alcoholic is a Drug Addict

Figure 54. The scientific temperance movement against alcohol, which had a strong Puritan influence, enacted alcohol prohibition in the United States. Image by The Scientific Temperance Foundation.

press, at the end of the decade, the United States decided to ban these substances. The first to do so was the state of California in 1966 when Ronald Reagan was governor, and they were later controlled at the federal level in 1969. Subsequently, in 1971, they were included in Schedule I of the International Convention on Psychotropic Substances, signed in Vienna, when Richard Nixon, the man who declared the so-called "war on drugs," was president of the United States.

In the 1980s, another of the world's most famous psychoactive substances, MDMA or ecstasy, came into vogue, being described as a semi-psychedelic and known for its entactogenic-empathogenic effects. It was banned in the United States in 1985 despite an administrative court recommendation to include it in Schedule III controlled substances, given that it is not very toxic and seemed to have psychotherapeutic effects. Despite pressure from some psychiatrists and other mental health professionals who used it for their treatments, the DEA (Drug Enforcement Administration) finally included it in its U.S. Schedule I classification, where the most dangerous substances with no recognized therapeutic value are placed, and in 1985 it was also included in Schedule I of the International Convention on Psychotropic Substances, which lists the most toxic and harmful substances considered to have little or no therapeutic value.

1.2 Criteria for Inclusion in One Control List or Another

Inclusion in one list or another does not always depend so much on the hazardousness or toxicity of the substance, or on its real therapeutic potential, but rather on a political or moral decision influenced by a given spatiotemporal context. In this regard, Nutt, King, and Phillips (2010) established a classification of the dangerousness of different drugs (legal and illegal) using a multitude of criteria, concluding that the least dangerous substances were psychedelic molecules, such as LSD and psilocybin, and semipsychedelics, such as cannabis and MDMA.[3] These substances were placed way below others, such as alcohol and tobacco, which, despite being more harmful, are legal.

In the words of an anonymous administrator and convention participant quoted by Mark Kleiman (professor of public policy and director of the Crime and Justice Program at New York University), ranking decisions are ultimately a consequence of the following premise: "If it's fun, it's Schedule One."[4]

1.3 The International Classification of Ketamine: A Substance with Recognized Medical Uses

The situation is different for ketamine, a substance with psychedelic and dissociative properties that was synthesized in 1962 by Calvin Stevens. Since then it has been used therapeutically in medicine and veterinary medicine as a general anesthetic and has also been included in the list of essential medicines of the World Health Organization (WHO) by

---

3. Nutt DJ, King LA, Phillips LD. 2010. Drug harms in the UK: a multicriteria decision analysis. The Lancet 376(9752):1558–1565.
4. Arbour, et al. 2019. (See full reference in note 2 of this appendix.)

virtue of its usefulness and safety. Since 2019, this substance, or rather one of its purified molecular forms (esketamine), patented by the pharmaceutical company Janssen (owned by Johnson & Johnson), has been recognized by the FDA and other drug agencies for the treatment of depression, and, likely, this therapeutic indication will also be extended to racemic (classic) ketamine—though this has not happened yet.

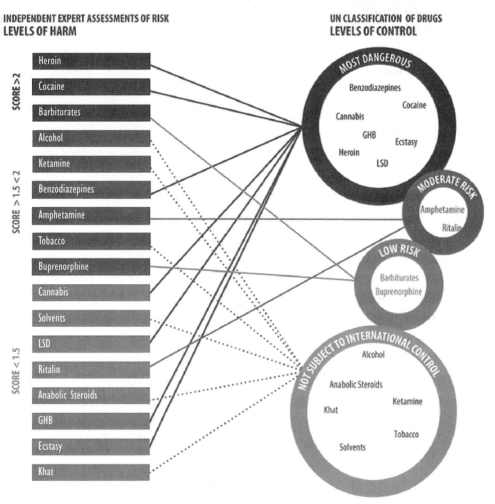

Figure 55. Levels of harm of different drugs as assessed by scientists, compared to their current international legal control levels. Figure adapted from: Nutt D, et al. 2007. Development of a rational scale to assess the harm of drugs of potential misuse. The Lancet 369 No. 9566:1047–53; Gomis B. 2016. Modernising Drug Law Enforcement. International Drug Policy Consortium, Drug Policy Guide, 3rd ed, 90–96.

Due to the rise of ketamine for recreational use, it was first controlled in the United States in 1999, and in 2006 it was listed by the United Nations Commission on Narcotic Drugs (CND) as a controlled substance under the 1971 Convention on Psychotropic Substances. Other states then transposed this prohibition into their national laws.

All the substances mentioned up to this point, except ketamine (which is in Schedule IV), are in Schedule I of the 1971 Convention on Psychotropic Substances where (according to the convention) the most dangerous and least valuable drugs in medicine are placed under control. Member states have also included them in the list where the most punishable substances under their respective national penal codes are to be found.

In the case of ketamine, this substance has always been recognized as having therapeutic properties as a general anesthetic and, more recently, as a psychiatric drug for the treatment of severe depression. For this reason, it has always been considered more therapeutic and less dangerous than other drugs; however, this cannot be considered scientifically correct since, for example, according to the report by Nutt et al., 2010, despite being below that of other legal drugs such as alcohol and tobacco, the harmful potential of ketamine for the individual and society is above that of LSD and psilocybin.

The WHO Expert Committee on Drug Dependence acknowledged that some concern had been expressed, stating:

> Placing ketamine under international control would have a negative impact on the availability and accessibility of this substance. This, in turn, would limit access to essential and emergency surgery, leading to a public health crisis in countries where no other affordable replacement anaesthetic is available.[5]

As can be seen, the case of synthetic drugs with psychedelic properties such as ketamine and MDMA or semisynthetic drugs such as LSD (derived from the ergot fungus) is not technically complicated when it comes to interpreting their legal status. As we will see below, legal

---

5. WHO. 2012. WHO Expert Committee on Drug Dependence, Report No. 35, Technical Report Series 973. Geneva (Switzerland): World Health Organization, 9.

interpretations become more complicated when dealing with plants or mushrooms that contain psychotropic controlled molecules.

The historical and legal arguments set out in the introduction to this appendix require us to navigate the paradoxical legislation and jurisprudence that regulate this issue.

2. States and Cities in the United States that Have Decriminalized the Use of Psychedelic Substances

2.1 U.S. Cities that Have Pioneered the Decriminalization of Psychedelic Substances

Since 2012, when the states of Colorado and Washington regulated access to cannabis for recreational use, there have been many efforts by associations advocating changes in current drug policies. To alleviate the great pandemic of mental illnesses that is increasingly present in society, such associations are seeking recognition of their therapeutic uses.

Thus, since then, not only has cannabis been regulated for recreational purposes in more than twenty states and Washington, DC, there have also been political and legislative movements to decriminalize the use of certain psychedelic substances in many parts of the United States, both at the state and municipal levels.

The first city to decriminalize the use of a substance other than cannabis was Denver, Colorado. In 2019, it did not quite legalize psilocybin (found in magic mushrooms), but it did, however, prohibit wasting police and judicial efforts to prosecute its use, thus being at the forefront of decriminalizing psychedelic drugs and recognizing their therapeutic value.

Other West Coast cities have also joined the reform, such as Oakland, California (historically very familiar with the use of entheogens), which in 2019 also decriminalized the use of plants, cacti, and mushrooms containing controlled substances such as psilocybin, mescaline, and DMT; and Santa Cruz, also in California, which in 2020 decriminalized the possession and cultivation of psilocybin-containing magic mushrooms, although the commercial sale of them remains illegal.

Washington, DC, followed suit in November 2020; and in 2021, the cities of Somerville, Bay State, and Cambridge, Massachusetts, did the same. Hence, we are no longer talking exclusively about cities on the West Coast. The decriminalization of psychedelics, like cannabis, has also reached the East Coast.

The latest cities to jump on the psychedelic bandwagon are Seattle and Port Townsend in Washington State; Arcata, Berkeley, Eureka, and San Francisco in California; Minneapolis in Minnesota; Evanston and Chicago in Illinois; Detroit, Ferndale, Hazel Park, and Ann Arbor in Michigan; Portland in Maine; Columbia in Maryland; and Amherst, Easthampton, Somerville, Northampton, Cambridge, and Salem in Massachusetts. These cities no longer prioritize the prosecution of crimes related to entheogenic plants. It, therefore, seems that, very soon, the possession and use of cannabis and other substances such as psilocybin (magic mushrooms) or mescaline (San Pedro cactus and peyote) will not be prosecuted in most states.

2.2 U.S. States that Have Decriminalized or Legalized the Use of Psychedelics

Regarding the decriminalization of psilocybin at the state level, the state of Oregon was the first to take the big step in November 2020, recognizing its use for therapeutic purposes, as it considers it useful for treating major depression and PTSD. Thus, possession of up to 12 g of magic mushrooms only entails a $100 fine or the completion of a health assessment. The possession of more than 12 g can lead to jail time. What is now completely legal in the state of Oregon is the provision of psilocybin treatments in specialized and certified centers. Colorado has decriminalized the personal use, possession, and private sharing of psilocybin and psilocin. This legislation also applies to the future inclusion of mescaline, ibogaine, and DMT, which will be considered for similar decriminalization after June 2026. However, retail sales of these substances are not allowed. The state plans to establish regulated "healing centers" where adults over the age of twenty-one can use these substances under professional supervision. These centers will offer a controlled environment for therapeutic use, but they are not set to begin operating until late 2024, with applications for licenses being accepted from that time.

The next state that seems to be getting ready to legalize the use of psilocybin for medicinal purposes is the state of California, where several proposals to legalize magic mushrooms' psychoactive molecule and other entheogenic plants for medicinal purposes have already been put forward. As of this writing, there are also such proposals in the states of New York, New Mexico, and New Jersey, and there are working groups studying legislative changes in at least ten other states.

2.3 Potential Problems Where U.S. Federal Law Comes into Play

Although these reforms are taking place at the local and state level, the United States is a federal republic, and U.S. federal law still includes psilocybin in its Schedule I controlled substances, which are considered the most dangerous and have the fewest therapeutic uses. This means that, even if they are in a city or state that has already decriminalized them if a person is caught in possession of these substances by FBI agents, they can be charged with possession of illegal drugs under U.S. federal law.

2.4 Conclusion

In summary, since some American cities don't consider them to be harmful and do instead consider them to have increasingly recognized therapeutic value, they are no longer prioritizing the efforts of their local police to prosecute people who use this type of drug. However, the only state that has legalized psilocybin for medicinal purposes is Oregon, and the U.S. Congress, which legislates at the federal level on drug issues, is not yet in favor of legalizing such substances. Therefore, the reader of this book should take special care if in possession of a certain quantity of substances considered psychedelic, as, with a few local exceptions, they are still prohibited nationally and, of course, internationally in all countries.

3. Graduation of Penalties for Trafficking and Use of Psychedelic Substances around the World

In order to impose a penalty on the offender, drug trafficking offenses in countries that follow the rule of law are usually classified based on three basic factors: the alleged dangerousness of the substance, the quantity seized, and the aggravating circumstances of the case.

3.1 Increased Penalties for the Dangerousness of the Substance

In order to assess the criminal risks that would exist in cases of arrest for possession or sale of these substances, it should first be checked whether or not the member state in question is signed on to the 1971 United Nations Convention, whether or not it has also transposed the convention into national law (i.e., whether such signed international convention has been "translated" into national law), and finally, whether those particular substances are controlled in any of the schedules of the national drug law of each state.

> Despite this, there are countries with analogue laws: the US Analogue Substances Act, enacted in 1988, which automatically bans a substance if its structure and effects are "substantially similar" to those of an already banned drug; or the UK's Psychoactive Substances Act of 2016, which by default bans any psychoactive substance that by stimulating or depressing the person's central nervous system . . . affects the person's mental functioning or emotional state.[6]

Penalties are usually imposed according to whether substances are more or less dangerous to public health. Some countries such as the United Kingdom classify them in Schedules A, B, or C, with the most (officially) dangerous substances such as cocaine, heroin, LSD, and psilocybin placed in Schedule A, amphetamines and cannabis in Schedule B, and tranquilizers in Schedule C. The United States also has five schedules, included in the first schedule those substances that are allegedly most abused, most toxic, and not medically licensed (LSD, psilocybin, DMT, and 2CB), with ketamine, for example, being included in Schedule III, given it is medically licensed.

---

6. United Kingdom. 2016. Psychoactive Substances Act. London: Crown, paragraph 2. Retrieved from the U.K. government website.

The case of Spain, for example, is more complex, having transposed the international drug conventions into domestic law by copying the same substances included in the schedules of the aforementioned international convention. Therefore, in the case of psychotropics, substances in Schedule I are officially more dangerous, and with less recognized therapeutic value, than those in Schedules II, III, and IV.

However, Article 36[7] of the Spanish Penal Code establishes a penal difference depending on whether or not the substance can cause serious damage to health. Paradoxically, however, this concept is not normative (not defined in the law), but jurisprudential (applied based on what previous judgments have interpreted), because the only drug currently classified by the jurisprudence of the Spanish courts as not causing serious harm to health is cannabis, and it is in Schedule I (the most controlled and with the least therapeutic potential) of the Spanish Narcotics Law 17/1967, while amphetamines and 2CB are in Schedule II (less controlled), although they are treated by case law as causing serious harm to health—yet another case of nonsensical legislation.

It should be noted that this jurisprudential concept, that of serious damage to health, is subject to change through the provision of pharmacological expert evidence, that is, what experts on the substance can say in court about its dangerousness. In fact, for example, MDMA (ecstasy) was considered by the Spanish National Court as a substance that does not cause serious damage to health in a hearing in 1994 in which the expert witness for the defense was Alexander Shulgin himself, considered the godfather or rediscoverer of this substance, as well as the mastermind behind the expansion of its use among the therapeutic community to treat post-traumatic stress disorder and other psychiatric illnesses. During the trial, the scientist compared MDMA to its chemical "big sister," MDA, to explain that MDMA is less neurotoxic than MDA and that it does not have high addictive power. Thanks to testimony, the court decided to consider ecstasy a substance that does not cause serious damage to health (Yoldi 1994) and

---

7. Yoldi J. 1994 Jan 23. El éxtasis no causa grave daño a la salud según la Audiencia Nacional [Ecstasy does not cause serious health effects, according to the National Court of Spain]. El País (Madrid). Spanish.

was therefore made punishable by a lesser penalty than cocaine and LSD. However, later on, Spanish court jurisprudence changed its opinion, considering ecstasy (MDMA) a health hazard. This was possibly due to the Leah Betts scandal, the eighteen-year-old British girl who died after taking an ecstasy pill at a house party with her parents. During the days when she was in a coma, a media campaign made the front page of newspapers in the United Kingdom and around the world, publishing photos of her on her deathbed and filling the streets up with pictures of her face accompanied by messages about the dangers of drugs. Later, the doctor who treated her said that she had died from overhydration, known as hyponatremia, as she drank too much water in an attempt to quash the effect of the pill. In reality, deaths from ecstasy use are not common and occur much less frequently than those related to alcohol or tobacco,[8] without resulting in the criminalization of their possession or distribution.

3.2 Increasing Penalties for Quantity Seized

The different countries that have banned the possession and sale of different psychedelic (or other) drugs also tend to establish tables to increase penalties according to the quantity of the substance seized.

This is the case, for example, in the United States, which has tables of equivalence between substances in which, if a certain quantity is exceeded, the minimum or maximum penalty required by federal law is increased. In the case of ecstasy, for example, there is a table of equivalence concerning cannabis, with the equivalence being 1–500. This means that 1 g of MDMA is equivalent to the penalty for 500 g of cannabis. This equivalence was raised in 2001 from 35–1 to 500–1, but in 2011, with the collaboration of the Multidisciplinary Association for Psychedelic Studies (MAPS), it was set by two American courts at 200–1, considering that the scientific reports provided in 2001 were based on exaggerated, and scientifically unsound, perceptions of the harmfulness of MDMA, and that MDMA was no more harmful than cocaine. In 2017, an attempt was made to reclassify the equivalence of ecstasy in a proceeding in which

---

8. Collin M. 2002. Estado alterado: la historia de la cultura del éxtasis y del acid house [Altered state: the history of ecstasy culture and "acid house"]. Barcelona (Spain): Alba Editorial. Spanish.

Dr. Rick Doblin, the founder of MAPS, was an expert witness, without succeeding in having the dangerousness of MDMA reconsidered.[9] However, with the work of people like Doblin and MAPS, MDMA is now in phase 3 clinical trials, and FDA recognition for the treatment of post-traumatic stress disorder and other psychiatric illnesses is expected by 2024.

3.3 Increased Penalties for Aggravating Circumstances

Penalties are also often increased for other aggravating circumstances, such as committing a crime with violence, belonging to a criminal organization, or trafficking minors.

Sentences for drug trafficking are typically set at between two and ten years in most countries, rising to twenty years or even life imprisonment in countries such as the United States or the United Kingdom, when there are very special and specific circumstances such as the use of criminal gangs or violence. There are regions where sentences can be particularly high, such as Africa, the Middle East, and Asia.

3.4 Tolerance in Cases of Small Quantities for Personal Use

In most European countries, some U.S. states, Canada, and in most South American countries, drug use for personal use is tolerated, and offenses for simple possession of drugs are usually punishable by a prison sentence of between six months and two years, which may be suspended if the offender is a first offender (no previous criminal record) or undergoing drug detoxification treatment. It might also just be replaced by a fine.[10]

However, the specific legislation in each country needs to be studied in detail to find out whether there is a law for minimum dose for personal use or whether simple possession is punishable by administrative fines and the like.

---

9. Multidisciplinary Association for Psychedelic Studies USSC Testimony re: MDMA March 15, 2017.

10. Cavada JP. 2020. Criterios para el sancionamiento del consumo o tráfico de drogas en el derecho extranjero [Criteria for the punishment of drug use or trafficking abroad]. Santiago de Chile: Biblioteca Nacional del Congreso de Chile. Spanish. Retrieved from the Biblioteca Nacional del Congreso de Chile website.

3.4.1 Latin American Countries

Latin American countries such as Colombia, Uruguay, Peru, and Mexico have minimum personal dose laws, in which small quantities of various substances cannot even be punished by an administrative rule.

In Peru, for example, drug trafficking is punishable by a sentence of eight to fifteen years, and possession for the purpose of trafficking is punishable by six to twelve years, and even life imprisonment if forced by violence or intimidation to plant drugs. However, possession for the personal use of up to 5 g of cocaine base paste, 2 g of cocaine hydrochloride, 8 g of marijuana, and 2 g of its derivatives, or 250 milligrams of MDMA or similar substances[11] is not criminalized. Having said this, it seems that the dose is seized even if it is not sanctioned in all countries except Uruguay.[12]

In Mexico and Colombia, for example, the constitutional courts have issued two rulings, on November 4, 2015, and June 6, 2019, respectively, in which, in the section on the weighing of affected fundamental rights and collective legal interests to be protected (public health and safety), it is concluded that these two collective interests should not prevail over the individual freedom and free development of the personality of the drug user, as long as the test of proportionality in the interpretation of these affected fundamental rights and protected legal interests is not passed. In other words, individual liberties prevail over the personal consumption of substances in the face of other considerations, such as public health and safety, allegedly threatened by personal drug consumption. However, the Colombian Constitutional Court had already declared the criminalization of drug use unconstitutional in Ruling C-221/94. Despite this ruling almost two decades ago, subsequent governments have criticized this judicial decision and attempted to recriminalize drug use for personal consumption, generating laws

---

11. Martín A, Muñoz J. 2019. El estatuto legal de la ayahuasca en España: la relevancia penal de los comportamientos relacionados con su consumo y posesión [Legal status of ayahuasca in Spain: the criminal relevance of behaviors related to its consumption and possession]. Valencia (Spain): Tirant lo Blanch. Spanish.

12. Salvo Uruguay, dosis mínima se incauta en toda A. Latina [With the exception of Uruguay, minimum doses are seized throughout Latin America]. El Nuevo Siglo (Bogotá, Colombia) 2018 Sept 6. Spanish.

that currently prohibit use but do not criminalize it. This ruling was used by academic researchers and by countries such as Switzerland and the Netherlands to adapt their arguments for their legislation.[13]

In Argentina, penalties range from one month to two years imprisonment, plus a fine for possession for personal use (Art. 14, second paragraph, Law 23.737); from one to six years imprisonment, plus a fine for simple possession (first paragraph of the same article); and from four to fifteen years imprisonment, plus a fine for possession for commercial purposes (5 inc. C of the same law). The latter Article 5 also establishes penalties for trafficking of four to fifteen years imprisonment, plus a fine, and some aggravating circumstances are described in subsequent articles. Cross-border trafficking is punishable under the Customs Code (Art. 866), with penalties ranging from four and a half months to sixteen years.

3.4.2 The Spanish Case

In Spain, as long as no specific quantities of psychedelics are found that exceed what is considered usual for daily personal use for three to five days, and provided there are no indications of trafficking (such as having the substance divided into doses, having a precision scale, a multitude of substances, a notebook with notes, cash, and so on), the case would not be sent to a criminal court. This has been established by the National Institute of Toxicology at a maximum of 2.4 g of pure MDMA or 0.003 g of LSD,[14] with a fine of between 601 and 30,000 euros[15] being imposed in these cases. However, this law is to be amended shortly, and it seems that fines for simple possession will be considered minor (the amount would be between 100 and 600 euros), and consumption on

---

13. Uprimny R. 2019. A 25 años de la sentencia C-221/94 en Colombia: una oportunidad perdida [Twenty-five years after the C-221/94 sentence in Colombia: a missed opportunity]. London: International Drug Policy Consortium. Spanish. Retrieved from the International Drug Policy Consortium website.

14. Instituto Nacional de Toxicología (2001). Informe sobre dosis mínima psicoactiva, de 18 de octubre de 2001 [Report on minimum psychoactive dose, October 18, 2001]. Madrid: Instituto Nacional de Toxicología. Spanish.

15. Ley Orgánica 4/2015, de 30 de marzo, de protección de la seguridad ciudadana [Organic Law 4/2015, March 30, on the protection of public safety]. Published in BOE [Official State Bulletin] No. 77, March 31, 2015. Spanish.

public roads will be punished with a fine of 601 euros.[16] However, perhaps because they are less prevalent in the population, substances such as psilocybin are not included in this table of quantities regarding personal consumption, nor do they appear in tables in other countries. In this case, and in order to calculate the dose that could be regarded as for personal use, and what quantities could be considered as trafficking and therefore subject to higher penalties, ad hoc expert evidence will be required. Despite exceeding the National Institute of Toxicology (INT) quantities, Spanish jurisprudence requires proof of intent to traffic the substance to convict through other evidence or indications.

To further highlight the lack of solid scientific criteria when establishing penalties for drug trafficking in Spain, we can recover this excerpt from an article on the words spoken by the director of INT at the time of issuing the famous report:

> "That table was part of a technical report that was sent in 2001 to the Supreme Court, but at no point did we address whether they should be used to set sentences or not," Gómez explained. Gómez agreed with the opinions of other experts consulted, and clarified that "the effect of a toxic substance on the organism depends on the person, their size, their state and how used to it they are. It is the same as with Valium which doesn't have the same effect on everyone. Some people fall asleep with one pill, others don't feel anything when they take two."[17]

In other words, not even the authors of the report considered it fair that sentences should be passed based on this technical report. As historically only a summary table has been available on the internet, I requested the report via Spain's Transparency Portal. It came as a great surprise to see that there were no bibliographical references that could

---

16. Azorín F. 2021 Dec 14. Reforma de la Ley Mordaza y cannabis: es urgente [Reform of the "Gag Rule" and cannabis: it's urgent]. El Salto (Madrid). Spanish.

17. Lázaro JM, De Benito E. 2004 Apr 11. Toxicología se desmarca del baremo que utiliza el Supremo para condenar a 'camellos' [Toxicology disassociates itself from the scale used by the Supreme Court to sentence "dealers"]. El País (Madrid). Spanish.

be refuted by other experts through contradictory expert evidence. Only a legend full of scientific and logical deficiencies could be found. For example, all substances have a range of daily doses, and to obtain the maximum amount for personal use, the highest end of the range is multiplied by 5 (in reference to five days of personal use). However, in the case of MDMA (ecstasy), it is stated that between one and fifteen tablets of 80 mg can be consumed per day when, according to the report, the norm is to take six tablets per day (which goes against the logic of the table, which always multiplies by 5 the highest dose of the range).

3.4.3 Personal Use Doses for Non-Scheduled Substances

In those cases where the substance in question does not appear in the table, it is up to the police to decide whether, depending on the dose seized, a case should be dealt with under criminal or administrative law. However, as we have said, the tables are not complete and do not cover the full range of psychopharmacological drugs used by people who consume illegal substances. In fact, in the case of psilocybin mushrooms, there is an acquittal in Spain that states the following:

> In the specific case of the ruling, 670 mushrooms weighing 202.5 grams were seized. In this sense, the minimum active dose [of pure psilocybin] is around 2 milligrams, 10 to 20 milligrams is a medium dose, and a high dose is 30 milligrams or more. The effects of medium doses last for 4 to 6 hours and those of high doses for up to 8 hours. Based on these parameters, the daily dose of [pure psilocybin] consumption can be put at around 100 mg. If we multiply this amount by 1.7 mg of psilocybin per mushroom, the result is just over 1 gram of this substance [pure psilocybin]. This is an amount that guarantees consumption for about 10 days.[18]

The reader will note, if experienced in the use of mushrooms, that, when it comes to psychedelics such as mushrooms or LSD, which are

---

18. Sentence from the Audiencia Provincial of Alicante No. 129/2013 February 28.
19. Legal situation of psilocybin mushrooms. Obtained from Wikipedia.

usually taken very infrequently, in annual or monthly doses at most, this ruling does not make much sense. However, drug jurisprudence is often constructed by people with little knowledge of the subject who assume that everyone who takes drugs is addicted and that taking a substance necessarily implies continuous use throughout the day to be under its effects twenty-four hours a day, every day. This flawed logic is probably derived from the problematic use of certain highly addictive opiates, such as heroin.

3.4.4 The Dutch Case

In the Netherlands, for example, possession of up to 5 g of fresh mushrooms and 0.5 g of dried mushrooms used to be tolerated, but in 2008, fresh mushrooms were explicitly banned. Previously, only dried mushrooms were considered to be "a preparation containing psilocybin" as defined by the 1971 Psychotropic Convention. Since 2008, the market switched from mushrooms to psilocybin-containing truffles, given that these fungal species were not explicitly controlled.[19]

3.4.5 Portugal and Its Risk and Harm Reduction Policy

Another country where possession of drugs for personal use is not criminalized is Portugal. Law 30/2000, adopted in November 2000 and enforced since July 2001, decriminalized the consumption, acquisition, and possession of drugs for personal use. A decree establishes the quantities that will not lead to criminal prosecution for each substance, estimating as a maximum the daily consumption of a drug for a period of ten days. If someone is caught consuming in the street, they are given the option of attending an interview with a committee comprised of a psychologist, a social worker, and a jurist so that they can analyze whether the situation is considered problematic consumption and, if so, offer the consumer therapeutic help (Cavada 2020).

3.4.6 France and Italy and Their Hardline Drug Policy

France, for its part, has always been a very belligerent country on drug issues within Europe. However, penalties for simple possession are less than one year, plus a fine, and the offender is usually required to attend and pay for a drug awareness course (Cavada 2020).

Italy is another country that establishes higher penalties for drug trafficking offenses, especially if committed by organized mafias. In terms of penalties for simple possession, it is also a rather tough country because, even if criminal proceedings are not initiated, serious administrative sanctions, such as the loss of one's driver's license, could be imposed. The country also offers substitution treatments for confiscations where no evidence of drug trafficking exists.[20]

3.4.7 Other European Countries
Concerning the tables of doses for personal use in other European countries, the European Union Drugs Agency (EUDA) produces summary tables for each country, available in the "Publications" section of the EUDA website ("Threshold quantities for drug offences").

3.5 Conclusion
In conclusion, in most countries that have a legal system based on the rule of law, with constitutions that protect and recognize fundamental rights of the individual, simple possession of drugs for personal use is not usually punishable by imprisonment. And if a prison term for personal use is stated in the law, it is usually symbolic and probably will be suspended if the person is a first offender or undergoes drug treatment. However, each factual situation can be interpreted in different ways, depending on the case, so to minimize the legal risks of possession and use, the drug user should do his or her part to understand how the supposed tolerance of personal possession for the personal use of drugs is interpreted in the legal practice of the relevant country.

3.6 Special Caution in Countries with Strict Drug Laws
In some countries around the world, especially in Africa, the Middle East, and Asia, what we in the West would call a "rule of law with due process and recognition of individual rights" is not strictly enforced. Therefore, drug possession in countries such as the Philippines, China, India, Malaysia, Qatar, Saudi Arabia, and others can lead to very seri-

---

20. Cavada JP. 2020. (See full reference in note 10 of this appendix.)

ous problems with the law. Paradoxically, it seems that Thailand,[21] one of these countries, intends to regulate recreational cannabis soon, having regulated access to the plant for medicinal purposes in 2020. It seems that drug policy is changing dramatically in some countries, and not necessarily only in Western ones or those with a democratic culture that, through the rule of law, recognizes the individual's fundamental rights.

4. International Control of Plants Containing Molecules Classified as Psychotropic under the 1971 Convention

As mentioned above, when we encounter interceptions of plant or fungal substances containing a molecule classified as psychotropic under the 1971 Convention on Psychotropic Substances, the legal interpretation becomes quite complicated.

4.1 The International Narcotics Control Board's Interpretation of the Conventions

In this section, we will analyze the thesis of the International Narcotics Control Board (INCB) when applying the international conventions to certain psychoactive plants that are not expressly controlled but contain substances that are.

The INCB or NCBI, in its 2010 and 2012 reports, states that there are only three plants controlled by the international drug conventions. These are only the cannabis plant (*C. sativa*); the coca leaf (*Erythroxylum coca*), from which cocaine is extracted; and the white poppy (*Papaver somniferum*), from which the opium needed to make morphine and heroin is extracted. In other words, the 1961 Convention on Narcotic Drugs only banned certain plants.

Although some active ingredients with stimulant or hallucinogenic effects contained in certain plants are controlled under the 1971 Convention, no plants are currently controlled under that convention

---

21. Tailandia, primer país de Asia que despenaliza la marihuana [Thailand, the first country to decriminalize marijuana]. Diario Las Américas (Miami, FL) 2022 Jan 25. Spanish.

or the 1988 Convention. Nor are preparations (e.g., decoctions for oral consumption) made from plants containing such active ingredients under international control.

Examples of such plants or plant materials are khat (*Catha edulis*), whose active ingredients cathinone and cathine are included in Schedules I and III of the 1971 Convention; ayahuasca, originating in the Amazon basin, mainly consisting of a preparation of *Banisteriopsis caapi* (a jungle vine) and another tryptamine-rich plant (*P. viridis*) that contains various psychoactive alkaloids such as DMT.[22]

No plants, even those containing psychoactive ingredients, are currently controlled under the 1971 Convention, although in some cases the active ingredients they contain may be under international control. For example, cathine and DMT are psychotropic substances listed in Schedule I of the 1971 Convention, while the plants and herbal preparations containing them, namely khat and ayahuasca, respectively, are not subject to any restriction or control measures.[23]

4.2 Possibility of Some Countries Controlling Certain Psychoactive Plants on an Individual Basis

Despite the explanation in the previous section, there may be countries that have expressly prohibited plants or parts of plants, as is the case in France and Italy with ayahuasca and in the Netherlands with magic mushrooms.

However, despite the interpretations of the International Narcotics Control Board, the truth is that, in most countries, seizures of ayahuasca are indeed reported and the police do usually confiscate magic mushrooms.

In Spain, most of the judicial precedents of criminal courts and provincial courts have considered that ayahuasca is not subject to the control regime of international treaties and that, therefore, its possession or sale is not criminally relevant, with some recent cases having resulted in acquittals and the return of the seized ayahuasca.

---

22. International Narcotics Control Board. 2011. 2010 Report. United Nations. New York.
23. International Narcotics Control Board. 2013. 2012 Report. United Nations. New York.

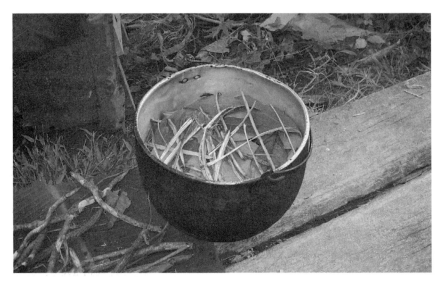

Figure 56. Ayahuasca, ready to be cooked. Photo by Terpsichore.

Thus, one of the latest court rulings, obtained by Francisco Azorín Ortega, the author of this appendix, states:

> To recapitulate, at the international level it seems clear that, either in its plant presentation or as a preparation (paradigmatically decoction for oral ingestion, which is the case here), ayahuasca cannot be understood to be included in the 1971 Convention, even though DMT is; and therefore, as a decoction or in its plant presentation (the plants from which it is obtained), it is not subject to international control.
>
> As a conclusion of this absence of specific mention at the national level and the lack of legal coverage in the 1971 Convention for its inclusion, we, therefore, understand that this preparation is not subject to special control in Spain, nor can it, therefore, be included in the definition of Article 368 of the Criminal Code.[24]

---

24. Sentence from the Provincial Court (Audiencia Provincial) of Málaga (Sección 1ª) No. 86/2021 March 10.

4.3 Pre-Trial Detention for False Positive Methamphetamine Tests

A person who was eventually acquitted for receiving a package with ayahuasca from Peru spent three months in prison because the substance showed a false positive for methamphetamine in the presumptive colorimetric test carried out by the police (something that usually happens with these plants). Therefore, until the substance was analyzed by a laboratory, with a confirmatory test, and until the corresponding appeals were filed because ayahuasca is not controlled, the investigated prisoner could not be released. Despite this, the antidrug prosecutor's office charged him with a crime against public health and asked for four years in prison.

There are also cases in which the investigating courts have ordered provisional imprisonment for the seizure of tobacco snuffs called rapé, sometimes containing DMT, which can show a false positive result for amphetamine or MDMA in the presumptive colorimetric tests carried out at customs. Even though a document from the Spanish Customs and Excise Department states that—even though almost all proceedings end in a file or acquittal and, normally, people who travel with suitcases loaded with ayahuasca from Colombia or Peru are no longer sent to provisional prison—controlled deliveries of ayahuasca should not be carried out, the truth is that as the appearance of these is that of a substance in greyish powder form that gives a false positive for MDMA, there have been provisional incarcerations for such rapés. In other words, if 3 or 4 kilos of rapés are seized and thus produce a false positive result, it is easy to be sent to prison until the health department determines, in a confirmatory manner, the substance in question and its quantification, an injustice that confirms the deficiencies of the system and the lack of public resources and knowledge when it comes to the state exercising its greatest power, the punitive power, or what the Romans called *ultima ratio* or the ultimate "reason of state": criminal law. Pretrial detentions have been criticized multiple times by the renowned criminal justice lawyer Gerardo Landrove Díaz as "legalized injustice."

5. Countries that Have Recognized or Banned Certain Plants with Controlled Molecules as Psychotropic

5.1 Lack of Clarity in the Wording of International Conventions

As mentioned above, the legal interpretation of the international accounting of plants containing molecules controlled as psychotropic by the 1971 Convention has never been simple or peaceful and has always generated controversy.

All this controversy stems from the wording of the international conventions and their official commentaries.

Sánchez and Bouso (2015) state in a report:

> What does not seem to be so clear is whether, in order to continue allowing the traditional use of these psychoactive plants, a state party to the convention must formulate a reservation or not. Reading the text of the treaty, one would say yes. But the commentary introduces a statement that, in a way, creates a paradox concerning what the convention itself establishes: when it says that ". . . Continued tolerance of the use of the hallucinogenic substances mentioned at the 1971 Conference does not require the formulation of a reservation under paragraph 4 of Article 32 since, following the traditional way of dealing with this issue in the framework of international drug control, the commentators consider that 'the inclusion in Schedule I of the active ingredient of a substance does not mean that the substance itself is also included in the Schedule if it is a substance clearly distinct from the substance which constitutes its active ingredient.'"

Therefore, there exists a disparity between the text of the convention and its official commentary signed by the U.N. Secretary-General. This discrepancy was clarified by the INCB in the above-mentioned reports of 2010 and 2012, which stated that these plants are not subject to international control.[25]

---

25. Sánchez C, Bouso JC. 2015. Ayahuasca: de la Amazonía a la aldea global [Ayahuasca: from the Amazon to the global village]. Barcelona (Spain): International Center for Ethnobotanical Education, Research, and Service. Spanish. Retrieved from the Transnational Institute website.

5.2 Countries that Have Made Exceptions to International Conventions and Rulings Clarifying This Issue

Only Mexico, Peru, the United States, and Canada have indeed made reservations to the 1971 international treaty to allow certain traditional uses of these substances by native communities in the Amazon basin or Indigenous reservations in the United States and Canada.[26]

In Chile, for example, a judgment was handed down in 2012 (Manto Wasi case) in which an ayahuasca ceremony had been infiltrated by a police officer. It was considered that ayahuasca could not be identified with DMT, controlled by the 1971 international convention and Decree No. 867 of 2007 of the Andean country controlling DMT, but that *P. viridis* and *B. cappi*, the individual plant components used to prepare ayahuasca, could be. The ruling stated that ayahuasca did not pose a danger to public health, and following the case, the director of public health requested that the Ministry of the Interior control ayahuasca. The initiative did not go forward.[27]

France, however, does follow a prohibitionist model. In 1999, a controversy arose over a complaint by a mother of a member of a daimist group[28] who claimed that her son had lost touch with reality. The case resulted in a conviction by the Paris Court of First Instance on January 15, 2004. The ruling was appealed to the Paris Court of Appeal, which ruled on January 13, 2015, that, although ayahuasca has hallucinogenic effects, it can be distinguished from synthetic DMT, which is what is undoubtedly subject to the prohibition under French law. Furthermore, it was not possible to speak of a preparation in the technical and legal sense, as this would require the existence of a pure substance. As a result, the court ruled in favor of acquittal (Martín and

---

26. Sánchez C, Bouso JC. 2015. (See full reference in note 25 of this appendix.)
27. Martín A, Muñoz J. 2019. (See full reference in note 11 of this appendix.)
28. Santo Daime is a syncretic spiritual practice that blends elements of Christianity with South American Indigenous traditions and African influences. Originating in the Brazilian Amazon in the 1930s, it was founded by Raimundo Irineu Serra, known as Mestre Irineu. Central to the Santo Daime religion is the sacramental consumption of ayahuasca, a psychoactive brew traditionally used by Indigenous peoples for spiritual and healing purposes.

Muñoz 2019). This pronouncement caused alarm among the authorities who, in order to avoid the situation highlighted in the ruling, decided to include all plants that are used or usually used in ayahuasca decoctions in the decree of April 20, 2005, thus prohibiting the uses of this plant in France (Martín and Muñoz 2019). Likewise, Italy banned ayahuasca in 2022.

5.3 Religious Uses and Cultural Heritage

In Brazil, a country with a strong "ayahuasca" culture, religious uses are recognized. Moreover, Brazil has not made a reservation to the 1971 Convention, and in 1985 the Ministry of Health included *B. cappi* and *P. viridis* as controlled substances. However, the "ayahuasca church," the União do Vegetal (UDV), fought a legal battle, which led to a study being carried out in communities that use ayahuasca in order to show that it had a significant positive effect (absence of alcoholism, lower infant mortality and malnutrition, crime rates close to zero, absence of violence, and the like). As a result of this report, the exclusion of plant species used in the preparation of ayahuasca was declared by Resolution No. 6 of February 4, 1986 (Martín and Muñoz 2019).

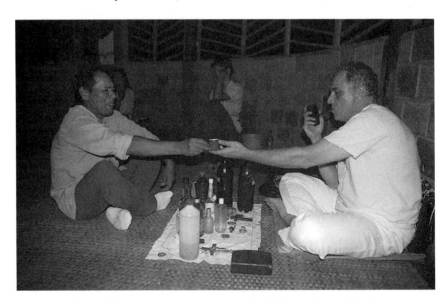

Figure 57. Ayahuasca ceremony at the Takiwasi Center (Peru).
Image by Takiwasi.

Subsequently, Resolution No. 1 of May 25, 2010, of CONAD (Council on Narcotic Drugs) ratified the legitimacy of the religious use of ayahuasca in one of the most detailed documents to date, regulating the uses of ayahuasca in religious practices, prohibiting its commercialization for profit, and emphasizing the avoidance of the offering in tourist packages (Martín and Muñoz 2019).

Peru, for its part, was the only country to make a distinction, under Article 32 of the 1971 Convention, regarding plants containing Schedule I psychotropic substances that have been traditionally used by certain small, clearly defined groups in religious ceremonies. This happened in 2008 when it declared ayahuasca a national cultural heritage. However, in contrast to Brazil, there is no detailed regulation, but rather a set of customs and practices.

Canada, the United States, and Colombia also allow religious uses of ayahuasca, and Canada and the United States also allow peyote cacti. In the Netherlands, religious uses of ayahuasca were allowed, but a Supreme Court ruling in 2019 changed the criteria and considered that the right to health prevails over religious freedom, declaring such use illegal.[29]

5.4 Attempts to Ban a Multitude of Medicinal Plants by the Spanish State

In 2004, an attempt was made in Spain to ban by ministerial order a list of 197 plants that were considered toxic or dangerous by the government at the time. The case was appealed before the Audiencia Nacional, which, as well as the Supreme Court in its ruling of July 9, 2008, nullified the ministerial order of January 28, 2004, on the grounds of formal errors in the order. The prohibition of these plants was not attempted again in Spain, so they are not subject to national control, or, as we saw earlier, to international control.

5.5 The Case of Peyote: Countries that Made Exceptions and Those that Consider It Illegal

Regarding peyote, a report by the ICEERS Foundation states: "There are more than forty North American Indian tribes in many

---

29. Ferrer I. 2019 Oct 2. El Supremo holandés prohíbe la importación de ayahuasca [Dutch Supreme Court bans the importation of ayahuasca]. El País (Madrid). Spanish.

parts of the United States and Canada that use peyote as a religious sacrament."

The psychoactive alkaloid in peyote, mescaline, is a controlled substance under the 1971 Vienna Convention and is included in Schedule I. Its use, sale, and manufacture are therefore prohibited. However, the peyote plant is not included in the schedules of the conventions, and its regulation depends on the legislation of each country. Thus, in Canada, mescaline is in Schedule III, and peyote is explicitly exempted from regulation if it is not prepared for ingestion, whereas in Brazil, France, Italy, and other countries, peyote is considered illegal. Other countries, such as Spain, do not mention peyote in the lists of controlled plants, although this does not imply that the sale of peyote cannot be considered an illegal act.

In the case of U.S. legislation, the use of peyote is permitted only in ceremonial contexts for persons belonging to the Native American Church.

> The Mexican government was one of the countries that, when adhering to the 1971 Convention and ratifying it on 20 February 1975, made an express reservation about its application, as there are certain Indigenous ethnic groups on its territory that traditionally use wild plants containing Schedule I psychotropic substances, including peyote. Within Mexican legislation, peyote cactus is not properly prohibited or regulated, as it is not included in any section of the General Health Law. Its use is permitted to the Huichols. Even so, peyote is considered an endangered plant, so, with exception of traditional use by Indigenous peoples, its collection is prohibited.[30]

6. Differences between Criminal Significance and Administrative Regulation of Plants Containing Molecules Classified as Psychotropic

To be fully aware of the legality surrounding these substances, it is necessary to differentiate between criminal and administrative legality. The

---

30. Peyote: basic information. Retrieved from the ICEERS website.

truth is that the uses of ayahuasca and other plants are not authorized at the administrative level in almost any country in the world. Only certain religious uses exist, as we have pointed out in the previous section. In other words, plants with controlled substances cannot be sold as food or medicine, even if they are not expressly prohibited by international conventions or national laws transposing these conventions into national law.

6.1 Projections for Recognition of Medical Use of Psychedelics in the Short Term

This lack of administrative recognition will be short-lived. Clinical trials with psilocybin, MDMA, LSD, ibogaine, and DMT are well advanced, and it is expected that the use of these substances will soon be authorized by the U.S., Canadian, European, and worldwide drug agencies for the treatment of depression, PTSD, anxiety, addictions, and other medical conditions. Just recently, in July 2023, Australia authorized the medical use of psilocybin and MDMA by licensed psychiatrists for patients with depression and post-traumatic stress disorder, respectively, provided they meet specific requirements.

6.2 The Canadian Case

Even though they are controlled, due to scientific advances in the recognition of the therapeutic properties of these molecules, their advanced clinical research stage into phases 2 and 3, the safety shown so far, and the need for new drugs in this field, given the delicate mental health situation exacerbated by the pandemic, the Canadian Health Agency (Health Canada) has just authorized doctors' access to psychedelic substances for mental health treatment.

In practice, this means that, in cases where other therapies have failed, are inadequate, or are unavailable in Canada, physicians are able, on behalf of patients with serious or life-threatening conditions, to apply for access to restricted medicines through Canada's Health Special Access Program (SAP).[31]

---

31. Canada Gazette, Part I, Volume 154, No. 50: Government Notices. 2020 Dec 12.

The proposed amendments are not intended to promote or encourage the early use of unapproved drugs, nor to circumvent well-established clinical trial or drug review and approval processes. However, these amendments could provide an additional potential option for physicians treating patients with serious or life-threatening conditions where other therapies have failed, are not suitable, or are not available.

As mentioned above, for the time being, ketamine or its isolate, esketamine, is the only substance that is currently fully administratively recognized. But very soon there will be more. Not only will cannabis be an administratively recognized medicine, but other, no less important substances (MDMA, psilocybin, DMT, and the like) are also knocking on the door to have their therapeutic properties recognized. One can already hear them: knock, knock!

In conclusion, the past and present research driven by people like Alexander Shulgin, Rick Doblin, Claudio Naranjo, David Nutt, Jordi Riba, Roland Griffiths, Amanda Fielding, José Carlos Bouso, Robin Carhart-Harris, the author of this book, and many others, will soon allow new substances, substances that have been unjustly stigmatized, demonized, abandoned, and banned for more than sixty years, to be authorized in order to deal more effectively with the pandemic of mental illness that plagues our societies.

7. Historical, Ecological, and Cultural Reasons Why Plants with Molecules Classified as Psychotropic Were Not Banned

7.1 Historical and Cultural Reasons

The historical, ecological, and cultural reasons for this choice are varied, but we could say that plants containing the alkaloid dimethyltryptamine (DMT) and mushrooms containing psilocybin are very numerous and are found all over the world. This means that legislators would have to control substances that could grow naturally in any field or garden patch.

One of the most important books ever written on psychedelics, *TiHKAL*, authored by two of the world's most influential people in the study of psychedelics, Alexander and Ann Shulgin,[32] contains a chapter titled "DMT Is Everywhere."

The chapter "Botany of Tryptamines" can be found within the third part of the book and at its beginning, we can read the following:

What is at the top of the pyramid? N,N-dimethyltryptamine, or DMT, of course. I think this is the right time to talk about the substance and the Drug Law, as 1966 is an interesting time when both stories converge. Manske first synthesised DMT in 1931. It was then independently isolated from two different plants: in 1946 by Goncalves de Lima (from *Mimosa hostilis*) and in 1955 by Fish, Johnson, and Horning (from *Piptadenia peregrina*). In 1956 Szára reported its activity in humans as a synthetic entity. The first legal restrictions on its research came in 1966 in response to the growing popularity it gained through the literature of Burroughs, Metzner, Leary, and others in the early 1960s; and in 1976, Christian noted its involvement as a component of the healthy human brain (and perhaps as a neurotransmitter).

The year 1965 marked the beginning of the use of initials, both as to substance and organisation names, in Federal Law Enforcement. It was then that, largely motivated by the psychedelic hippie movement of the younger generation at the time, the Drug Abuse Control amendments were passed and came into force. This led to the founding of the BDAC (Bureau of Drug Abuse Control), which became part of the FDA. These amendments were drafted to try to control non-narcotic substances (so-called dangerous substances) such as DMT, LSD, DET, ibogaine, bufotenine, DOM, MDA, MDMA, and TMA. BDAC was an agency that acted in parallel, but not in contact, with the already existing FBN (Federal Bureau of Narcotics), which was exclusively dedicated to the control of the three known narcotic substances: heroin, cocaine, and marijuana. . . .

---

32. Shulgin Alexander, Shulgin Ann. 1997. TiHKAL: the continuation. Berkeley (CA): Transform Press.

Therefore, the origin of the control of DMT as a pure substance comes from factors such as in synthesized onion, in both its pure and crystallized form, given it was synthesized even before it was discovered within countless plants, as well as to the fact that it is even found in the human brain, something that should not be so surprising given its similarity to the serotonin molecule and hence its metabolic proximity.

7.2 Ecological Reasons

A little further on, Shulgin and Shulgin (1997) continue: "The answer to the second question is that DMT is simply almost everywhere you look. It is in this flower here, in that tree there, and in those animals further away."

The book's chapter is divided into sections to indicate where DMT can be found: marine world (*S. ehina*, *S. auria*, etc.); toads (*Bufo*); herbs (birdseed or *Phalaris* species, etc.); legumes (*Acacia*, *Mimosa*, Illinois flower, *Sophora secundiflora* seed or mescal bean, etc.); *Psychotria* (*P. viridis*); limes, lemons, and Angostura bitters (*Zanthoxylum arborescens* and *Z. procerum*) (Shulgin and Shulgin 1997).

Different species of psilocybe mushrooms also grow wild around the world, as can be seen in various books. Many sources can be

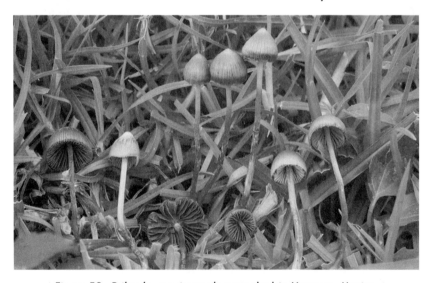

Figure 58. *Psilocybe mexicana* photographed in Veracruz, Mexico.
Image by Alan Rockefeller.

consulted to accredit the large number of mushrooms containing molecules that are controlled under international law (psilocin and psilocybin), but some notable ones are the following: *Psilocybin Mushrooms of the World*,[33] *Psilocibes (The Mushrooms)*,[34] *Teonanácatl*,[35] and *Pharmacotheon*.[36] Almost all varieties of psilocybin mushrooms discovered up to the time of publication can be consulted here.

In the book *Psilocibes*, we find chapter four, authored by Oscar Parés, which lists some of the existing varieties of mushrooms that contain psilocybin: *cubensis, Panaeolus/Copelandia cynescens,* and *Panaeolus/Copelandia tropicalis.*

The author states:

There is a third grouping of psilocybin fungi that is worth considering. It is not distinguished from the previous two by its genetic family but by its form or presentation. Called truffle (Latin: *sclerotium*, plural: *sclerotia*), it is a hardened compact mass of mycelium containing psilocybin. It is produced when the environmental conditions are not favourable for the flower, or reproductive apparatus (read: the fungus) to sprout from the long underground mycelium. Under this heading, we would include the most widespread *Psilocybe tampanensis*, but sclerotia of *Psilocybe mexicana* and *Psilocybe atlantis* are also commercially available.

7.2.1 Psilocybe Fungi Found on the Iberian Peninsula

Following the quotation in the previous section:

Psilocybe cyanescens and *Copelandia cyanescens* are also known to have been found in open fields on the Iberian Peninsula. . . .

---

33. Stamets P. 1996. Psilocybin mushrooms of the world: an identification guide. Berkeley (CA): Ten Speed Press.
34. Bouso JC, editor. 2013. Psilocibes: the mushrooms. Motril (Spain): Ultraradio.
35. Ott J, Bigwood J, Wasson G, Belmonte D, Hoffmann A, Weil A, Evans R. 1985. Teonanácatl: hongos alucinógenos de Europa y América del Norte [Teonanácatl (flesh of the gods): hallucinogenic mushrooms of Europe and North America]. Madrid: Swan. Spanish.
36. Ott J. 1996. Pharmacotheon. Barcelona (Spain): La Liebre de Marzo.

We now turn to two other psilocybe fungi of special interest that occur in the Iberian context. The first of these is *Psilocybe hispanica*. This fungus was discovered in the Huesca Pyrenees.

In Galicia, we find the *Psilocybe gallaeciae*, which according to Guzmán, one of the most prestigious mycologists in the world, belongs to the variety *P. mexicana*. There are indications that two other mushrooms with psilocybin content can be found in Catalonia: *Psilocybe subbalteatus* and *Panaelus cyanescens*.

The book we have just quoted also contains a chapter titled "Visionary Fungi" in the Iberian Peninsula, written by Ignacio Seral Bozal.

To get an idea of the number of psychoactive mushrooms that are not legally controlled and exist in the Iberian Peninsula, we will cite the different sections into which this chapter is divided such as we previously did with the *TiHKAL* chapter.

- *Amanita muscaria*.[37] Species: *A. phantherina* and *A. gemmata*.
- Genus *Panaeolus*. Species: *P. cyanescens*.
- Genus *Pluteus*. Species: *P. salicinus* and *P. antricapillus*.
- Genus *Inocybe*. Species: *I. aemacta*, *I. corydalina*, *I. coelestium*, and *I. aeruginascens*.
- Genus *Gymnopilus*. Species: *G. spectabilis*.
- Genus *Psilocybe*. Species: *P. hispanicae*, *P. galicae*, *P. cyanescens*, and *P. semilanceata*.

As we can see, the argument put forward to defend the noncontrol of plants with DMT content is also applicable in the case of psilocybe mushrooms. There are many genera and species of psychoactive mushrooms in the world. Some of them, such as *A. muscaria*, do not even contain controlled molecules. Ibotenic acid and muscimol (the psychoactive ingredients of this species) are not subject to international control; therefore, in this case, it would not even raise doubts regard-

---

37. Psychoactive but not psychedelic mushroom.

ing varieties of mushrooms that contain controlled molecules that we are trying to resolve. Despite this lack of regulation, the consumption of this mushroom does not produce classic psychedelic effects and actually poses far more health risks than any other psilocybin-containing fungal species.

Bearing this in mind, in the case of a hypothetical control of these mushrooms, one could present the exception of the international convention that states that if the organism grows wild in that territory and there is a traditional use, reservations to the convention could be accepted.

Mescaline-containing cacti are also present not only in American countries but also in Spain and other southern European countries.

7.3 Reasons Given in the 2014 TNI Report

To understand a little more about how these international conventions were put together, let us quote a paragraph from a TNI report (Transnational Institute 2014):

> The problem regarding how to deal with the traditional uses of certain plants arose again at the 1971 Conference, especially concerning psilocybin-containing mushrooms and the mescaline-containing peyote cactus, both hallucinogenic substances listed in the 1971 Convention schedules. Then, as of now, mushrooms and peyote were used in religious and healing ceremonies by Mexican and North American Indigenous groups. Unlike the position they took during the 1961 negotiations, this time the US authorities accepted the "consensus that it is not worth trying to impose control measures on biological substances from which psychotropic substances can be obtained . . . North American Indians in the United States and Mexico use peyote in religious rites and the misuse of this substance is considered sacrilege." By excluding plants from which alkaloids could be extracted from the scheduled lists, the 1971 Convention deviated, with good reason, from the prevailing zero-tolerance rule that had been applied in the Single Convention [on Narcotic Drugs]. The very concept of "psychotropic substances"

was a distortion of the logic underpinning the control framework, as the term lacks scientific credentials and was originally invented, in effect, as an excuse to avoid the much stricter controls of the Single Convention being applied to the wide range of psychoactive, mostly synthetic, drugs included in the 1971 Convention.[38]

7.4 Conclusion

There may be several reasons as to why no plants are controlled under the 1971 Convention on Psychotropic Substances. One of the most likely reasons is the fact that if all plants containing any active substances categorized as a psychotropic were to be banned, a large part of the world's flora would be illegal. Given that in some other instances some plants are indeed controlled, it may also be that the conventions understand that it is not desirable to control plants that are not considered extremely dangerous. After all, unlike controlled plants such as the opium poppy or the coca plant, which could kill in high doses, psychedelic plant sources rarely pose a direct risk to physical health.

In conclusion, it seems that solid arguments exist such as mental health, risk and harm reduction, and what is known as the "management of risks and pleasures," and not only on a scientific but also on a historical, legal, cultural, and ecological level. These arguments can and should be taken into account by both the readers and public authorities when, with the greatest legal guarantees, facilitating access to psychedelic therapy.

---

38. Henman A, Metaal P. 2014. Hora de abrir los ojos [It's time to open our eyes]. Amsterdam (The Netherlands): Transnational Institute. Spanish.

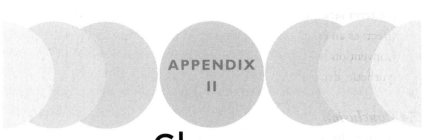

APPENDIX II

Glossary

ACTION POTENTIAL: An electrical discharge wave that travels along the axonal cell membrane modifying its electrical charge distribution. Its generation begins with the detection of neurotransmitters by receptors and ends with the release of the neurotransmitter from the axon terminal.

ALKALOIDS: Secondary plant metabolites, usually synthesized from amino acids, which have in common their water solubility at acidic pH and their solubility in organic solvents at alkaline pH. True alkaloids are derived from an amino acid and are therefore nitrogenous. All those with the amine or imine functional group are basic. Many psychoactive substances are alkaloids.

AMYGDALA: A subcortical structure located in the inner part of the medial temporal lobe whose main function is to integrate emotions with the corresponding response patterns.

ANGULAR GYRUS: Brain area where the temporal lobe, occipital lobe, and parietal lobe converge, as well as the executive frontoparietal network, the ventral attentional network, and the default mode network.

ASSOCIATION CORTEX: Areas of the cerebral cortex where different types of information (motor, limbic, sensory) are integrated.

AUTISM: A broad spectrum of disorders characterized by persistent impairments in communication and social interaction in a variety of contexts, coupled with restrictive and repetitive patterns of behavior, interests, or activities.

AUTONOMIC NERVOUS SYSTEM: The part of the nervous system that controls involuntary actions, such as heart rate, respiratory rate, blood pressure, sweating, dilation, and contraction of blood vessels.

AXON: Neuronal projection that transmits an electrical current, called an action potential, to signal the release of neurotransmitters.

AXON TERMINAL: The end of the axon where the vesicles with the neurotransmitters are located and released to the extracellular space.

AYAHUASCA: Amazonian cocktail of plants that, according to some indigenous communities, has medicinal properties. Although the content may vary from one preparation to another, this cocktail is based on the plant *Banisteriopsis caapi* and often includes *Psychotria viridis*, where DMT is found.

BIPOLAR DISORDER: A mental disorder that causes fluctuating and often extreme changes in mood, energy, activity level, and concentration; fluctuating between depressive and euphoric states. Formerly known as manic depressive psychosis.

BOTTOM-UP INFORMATION: Information going from lower orders of integration to higher orders of integration.

BRAIN WAVES: Rhythmic patterns of electrical activity produced by the brain.

CEREBRAL CORTEX: Outermost structure of the brain, organized vertically in columns and horizontally in layers.

CHANNEL: Transmembrane proteins that allow the passage of ions across a cell membrane.

CLASSIC PSYCHEDELICS: Psychedelics that act through the serotonin 2A receptor such as LSD, psilocybin, and DMT.

COMPLEXITY: Property of complex systems whose behavior is unpredictable and whose state is highly sensitive to initial conditions.

CONNECTIVITY: Communication between different areas of the brain as measured by the degree of correlation between the activity of the different areas concerned.

CONNECTIVITY MAP OF AREA X: When studying the areas that are highly connected to a particular area (area X), the set of brain areas that are highly synchronized with it.

CONTROL GROUP: In research, a group that, without receiving the drug or intervention investigated in a particular study, is subjected to the same experimental conditions as the group that does receive the drug or intervention.

CRIMINAL SIGNIFICANCE: When an alleged offense is covered by an article of the criminal code of a given state and the consequence is a legal measure consisting of a custodial sentence, a financial penalty, or the deprivation of a fundamental right, such as disqualification from holding public office, disqualification from participating in elections, or disqualification from association with the victim. There are also security measures consisting of the internment of persons who are not criminally liable, such as those who have committed the offense because of a psychiatric illness.

DAIMISTA: Parishioner of the Church of Santo Daime (ayahuasca church).

DEA: Drug Enforcement Administration. It is the agency of the U.S. Department of Justice dedicated to combating the smuggling and use of illegal drugs in the United States, as well as money laundering. Although it shares jurisdiction with the FBI, domestically, along with U.S. Immigration and Customs Enforcement and U.S. Customs and Border Protection, it is the sole agency responsible for coordinating and prosecuting antidrug investigations abroad.

DEFAULT MODE NETWORK: A functional network at the top of the integration chain and highly involved in processing information from within the system, related to memory and emotion and combining it with highly processed information from outside. Highly involved in generating a sense of identity and social cognition.

DENDRITE: Neural projection responsible for receiving signals from the extracellular space via receptor proteins located in its membranes.

DEPRESSION: A mental disorder characterized by low self-esteem and mood, lack of motivation and energy, and intrusive and negative thoughts defined as rumination.

DESIGNER DRUG: Engineering in the synthesis of new drugs whose mission is to create substances that mimic other substances under international or national control. The classic example of a designer drug would be fentanyl, which mimics controlled opiates. And the paradigm of a psychedelic designer drug would be 2CB, synthesized by A. Shulgin in 1974 in an attempt to find a molecule similar to mescaline. Terms such as NPS (new psychoactive substance) or RC (research chemicals) are also used to define these when they are very new and not yet internationally controlled.

DETOXIFICATION TREATMENT: A measure imposed by a court as a substitute for a prison sentence for drug-related offenses. The convicted person must complete the treatment under the warning that, if they fail to attend the appointments, or fail to complete the treatment, the benefit of the suspended sentence will be revoked.

DMT: A psychoactive molecule widely distributed in nature that can be vaporized, injected intravenously, or ingested. To obtain psychoactive effects in the latter case, it is necessary to additionally consume a substance that inhibits an enzyme in the stomach that degrades it.

DOPAMINE: A neurotransmitter heavily involved in motivation and addiction, produced by neurons in the substantia nigra and ventral tegmental area.

DORSOLATERAL PREFRONTAL CORTEX: Area of the prefrontal cortex par excellence, involved in executive processes such as short-term working memory.

EEG (ELECTROENCEPHALOGRAM): A technique that detects electrical activity in the brain using small metal discs (electrodes) attached to the scalp.

EGO DISSOLUTION: Loss of the perception of separation between the "self" and the world.

EMPATHOGENS: Molecules like MDMA that promote feelings of empathy and prosocial behavior, mainly through the release of serotonin. Also referred to as entactogens.

ENZYMES: Organic molecules that accelerate the speed of relevant chemical reactions.

EUROPEAN UNION DRUGS AGENCY (EUDA): A European public agency set up to monitor and publish reports on the prevalence of drug use in the states of the European Union and to assess and advise on drug policy.

EXECUTIVE PROCESSES: Goal-directed cognitive abilities. They influence our behaviors, through self-regulation, and cognitive and emotional activity, by selecting which information should be processed according to the goal. The functional network involved in these processes is the frontoparietal control network, which contains the dorsolateral prefrontal cortex.

FEDERAL LAWS: Laws passed in the U.S. Congress. They differ from the laws of individual states in that they affect all American citizens and can only deal with certain very important competencies attributed by the U.S. Constitution to the U.S. Congress, located on Capitol Hill in Washington, DC. The FBI (Federal Bureau of Investigation) is responsible for investigating offenses covered by and punishable under federal law.

FRACTAL: Geometric object whose basic structure, fragmented or apparently irregular, is repeated at different scales.

FRONTAL LOBE: Cerebral lobe containing the primary motor cortex responsible for sending projections that activate muscles.

FRONTOPARIETAL CONTROL NETWORK: Functional network involved in executive processes. Contains the dorsolateral prefrontal cortex.

FUNCTIONAL MAGNETIC RESONANCE IMAGING (fMRI): A neuroimaging technique used to explore the functionality of different parts of the brain by indirectly measuring the activity of these areas by detecting changes in oxygen consumption.

GABA (GAMMA-AMINOBUTYRIC ACID): Main inhibitory neurotransmitter in the brain.

GAIA: According to the Gaia hypothesis, devised by James Lovelock (1919–2022), the atmosphere and the surface of planet Earth behave as a system where life, its characteristic component, is responsible for self-regulating its essential conditions, such as temperature, chemical composition, and salinity, in the case of the oceans. Gaia would behave as a complex, self-regulating system, tending toward equilibrium.

GLUTAMATE: The most abundant excitatory neurotransmitter in the brain.

GLUTAMATERGIC: A neuron that transmits information by releasing glutamate.

HETERODIMER: Heterodimers are formed when two different receptors bind and begin to act together producing a new intracellular cascade of information.

HETEROMODAL AREA: Areas that process information from several senses.

HIERARCHICAL PREDICTIVE CODING: Theory that postulates that the brain forms a model of the world, which it uses to predict incoming information, and, by taking into consideration the discrepancies between this incoming information and the predictions made by the model, generates prediction errors through which it updates the model.

HIPPOCAMPUS: Phylogenetically ancient subcortical structure, heavily involved in memory encoding and recollection, working closely with the amygdala.

HYPOTHALAMUS: An area of the brain that is part of the limbic system. Acts as the interface between the nervous system and the endocrine system. It plays an important role in the regulation of emotions, as well as being the main hormonal regulator. Depending on the information it receives from the amygdala, it releases certain hormones into the bloodstream.

ICEERS FOUNDATION: A nonprofit foundation based in the Netherlands and Spain dedicated to the research of applications of plants containing psychoactive molecules, controlled or not, for the treatment of different diseases, as well as to the protection of the cultures that use them in a traditional way. They have ECOSOC status at the United Nations Commission on Narcotic Drugs.

INSIGHT: A moment of profound revelation that reshapes the way we look at and understand something, often offering a solution to a problem.

INSULA: Brain structure involved in limbic and cognitive processes.

INTEGRATION: Refers to the process by which different information from lower levels converges at higher levels to give rise to conscious experience.

INTERNATIONAL CONVENTION ON PSYCHOTROPIC SUBSTANCES: Together with the 1961 Single Convention on Narcotic Drugs and the 1988 United Nations Convention against Illicit Traffic in Narcotic Drugs and Psychotropic Substances, the 1971 Convention forms the current international drug control system. It was prompted by the rise in the use of hallucinogenic or psychedelic drugs and to control nonnarcotic substances, such as those included in the 1961 Convention.

INTERNATIONAL NARCOTICS CONTROL BOARD, INCB (NCBI): An independent, quasi-judicial body of experts established under the 1961 Single Convention on Narcotic Drugs by the merger of two bodies, namely the Central Standing Committee on Narcotic Drugs, established under the 1925 International Opium Convention, and the Narcotics Control Bureau, established under the 1931 Convention for Limiting the Manufacture and Regulating the Distribution of Narcotic Drugs. INCB consists of thirteen members, each elected to serve for a term of five years by the Economic and Social Council.

ION: An atom with an electrical charge that can be either positive (cation) or negative (anion).

JURISPRUDENCE: Doctrine established repeatedly by the Supreme Court or the Constitutional Court when interpreting the constitution and its laws.

LEGISLATION: A set of rules and laws that regulate the relations between people in a country or a particular sector. Legislation makes it possible to organize a given sector and a country as a whole.

LIMBIC NETWORK: Functional cortical network involved in memory and emotions. The regions that comprise it receive information from the limbic relay nucleus of the thalamus.

LIMBIC SYSTEM: A collection of various brain structures located subcortically and cortically. It is formed by phylogenetically ancient structures and is primarily responsible for affective information.

LSD (LYSERGIC ACID): Psychedelic molecule discovered by Albert Hofmann in 1943.

MAPS (MULTIDISCIPLINARY ASSOCIATION FOR PSYCHEDELIC STUDIES): A nonprofit organization founded in 1984 by Rick

Doblin to research the medical and cultural uses of psychedelic substances.

MDMA: 3,4-Methylenedioxymethamphetamine, a pseudopsychedelic, empathogenic, and entactogenic molecule first synthesized in 1912 by Merck Laboratories and rediscovered in the mid-1970s by chemist Alexander Shulgin. Currently used mainly in clinical trials with patients suffering from post-traumatic stress disorder. Common names: ecstasy and molly.

MEDIAL: Plane of the brain between the two hemispheres, as opposed to lateral.

MEDIAL TEMPORAL LOBE: Medial area of the temporal lobe containing phylogenetically ancient structures involved in memory.

MEG (MAGNETOENCEPHALOGRAM): A noninvasive technique that measures the magnetic fields produced by electrical currents in the brain. It uses a kind of helmet, in which the head is inserted and which contains sensors capable of detecting the magnetic fields associated with the electrical currents of neuronal axons.

MESSENGER RNA: RNA strand used to synthesize a protein.

META-ANALYSIS: A statistical technique that combines and summarizes the results of several similar individual studies.

MINDFULNESS: Meditative state of mind based on attention to the present moment and nonjudgment.

MINISTERIAL ORDER: A legal instrument of Spanish law that is not strictly speaking a law, decree, or regulation, and which serves, in this case, to include substances in one or another list of the different national drug laws that transpose international conventions into domestic law.

MNEMONIC: In reference to memory processes.

NARCOTIC SUBSTANCES: These are the substances included in the 1971 Convention on Psychotropic Substances. This is a legal or juridical term that includes those substances in Schedules I and II of the 1961 Convention on Narcotic Drugs. Moreover, many of those included in this book could not be defined as narcotic drugs, but cannabis would also be defined as hallucinogenic, or semipsychedelic. And cocaine, which is not a narcotic in a strict sense, can be considered as a local anesthetic with stimulant properties.

NEUROGENESIS: Creation of new neurons.

NEURON: Cell of the nervous system.

NEUROPLASTICITY: Strengthening or weakening of previous synapses, as well as the formation of new synaptic boutons, dendrites, axons, and even new neurons.

NEUROTRANSMITTER: Molecule that controls and transmits information from a neuron to target cells throughout the body. These may be another neuron, a muscle cell, or a gland.

NORADRENALINE: Molecule that can act as a neurotransmitter or as a hormone. In the nervous system it is released from the locus coeruleus and is involved in maintaining appropriate alertness.

OCCIPITAL LOBE: Cerebral lobe containing the primary visual cortex.

ORBITOFRONTAL CORTEX: Area of the prefrontal cortex highly connected with the limbic system and involved in the control of impulses and emotions.

ORDER OF INTEGRATION: The level of integration of information at a given location. In relation to a specific area, there are higher orders and lower orders.

PARAHIPPOCAMPAL CORTEX: Phylogenetically ancient cortical area, located in the medial part of the temporal lobe, highly involved in memory recollection and encoding.

PARIETAL LOBE: Cerebral lobe containing the primary somatosensory cortex.

PET (POSITRON EMISSION TOMOGRAPHY): A functional imaging technique that uses radioactive markers to obtain information about where and how a particular metabolic process is taking place within the body.

PLACEBO: An inactive substance, or other intervention, that looks like and is administered in the same way as the active drug or treatment being tested. The effects of the active drug or other intervention are compared with the effects of the placebo, which is consumed by the control group.

POSTERIOR CINGULATE CORTEX: Highly associative area of the brain that is part of the default mode network.

POST-TRAUMATIC STRESS DISORDER (PTSD): A mental health disorder triggered by the experience of a terrifying and traumatic situation.

PREDICTION ERROR: A signal that is generated when incoming information from lower levels of integration does not match the information contained in the model at higher levels.

PREDICTIVE CODING: Same as hierarchical predictive coding above.

PREFRONTAL CORTEX: Area of the frontal lobe involved in planning, selecting, and executing actions. The prefrontal cortex represents the later evolved part of the prefrontal lobe.

PRESUMPTIVE COLOR TEST: A field test performed by the police to provide a quick indication that a particular substance may be classified as a narcotic or psychotropic substance. It differs from confirmatory tests in that, in presumptive tests, there is a possibility of false positives and negatives, and it is not possible to quantify the purity of the substance seized and, therefore, whether it exceeds the minimum psychoactive dose, or whether it is a toxic dose. Examples of a presumptive test: Duquenois or Marquis.

PRIMARY SENSORY CORTEX: Areas of the cerebral cortex where sensory information is initially received.

PROPORTIONALITY TEST: Legal doctrine for the interpretation of conflicting fundamental rights in a legal relationship, whether these concern two fundamental rights of the individual, or a right of the individual as opposed to collective legal goods, such as public health or collective security.

PSILOCYBIN: Psychedelic molecule found in *Psilocybe* mushrooms.

PSYCHEDELIC: A molecule capable of abruptly altering the state of consciousness. Classic psychedelics act through the serotonin 2A receptor. Some classifications consider MDMA a psychedelic, but not a classical psychedelic. Others prefer to consider MDMA an empathogen or a pseudopsychedelic.

PSYCHEDELIC SESSION: Psychoactive session, within psychedelic-assisted therapy, in which the patient consumes the psychedelic molecule accompanied by music and psychotherapists.

PSYCHOSIS: A delusional state of mind in which there is a loss of contact with reality.

PSYCHOTROPIC SUBSTANCES: Those included in the 1971 Convention on Psychotropic Substances. As with narcotic drugs, this is a legal term for such substances that can be classified as stimulants (amphetamine) or hallucinogens (LSD).

RECEPTOR: Membrane protein that is responsible for detecting neurotransmitters on the outside of the neuron and, by changing conformation, activating a response to them that triggers a cascade of intracellular changes that modify the neuronal interior.

REGULATION: A rule that develops the content of a law.

RELAY NUCLEUS: Unimodal thalamic nuclei with nondiffuse projections (as opposed to nonspecific thalamic nuclei), specialized in processing a particular type of information (as opposed to the association thalamic nuclei).

RESERVATION TO AN INTERNATIONAL TREATY: A unilateral act by which a State or an international organization expresses its intention to exclude or modify an obligation arising from an international treaty.

REUPTAKE PROTEIN: A type of transport protein located in the axon terminal membrane. It is responsible for reintroducing the neurotransmitter released by the presynaptic neuron into the synaptic cleft back into the presynaptic neuron.

SECOND SUMMER OF LOVE: A social phenomenon between 1988 and 1989 in the United Kingdom during which acid house music developed, providing the soundtrack for the emergence of the rave culture, a synergistic combination of a drug (namely ecstasy, where it was also known as "E") together with another way of understanding music recreationally through group dance.

SEMANTICS: The study of various aspects of the meaning, sense, or interpretation of linguistic signs such as symbols, words, expressions, or formal representations.

SEROTONIN: A neurotransmitter that is heavily involved in mood regulation produced by neurons in the raphe nuclei.

SEROTONIN REUPTAKE INHIBITORS (SSRIs): The most widely used antidepressants. They act by increasing the concentration of serotonin in the synaptic space through preventing its re-entry into the axon terminal by blocking the neurotransmitter's reuptake transporter proteins located in the axon terminal membrane.

SHAMAN: Intermediary between the visible world and the spirits with whom, in a trance-like state, they communicate for guidance or healing.

SHAMANISM: A set of beliefs based on the premise that the visible world is permeated by invisible forces and spirits from parallel dimensions that coexist simultaneously with ours and affect all manifestations of life.

SINGLE CONVENTION ON NARCOTIC DRUGS: The international treaty signed on March 30, 1961, in New York, which forms the international legal framework for drug control. The convention defined narcotic drugs as "any of the substances in Schedules I and II, natural or synthetic," and recognizes in its preamble that the medical use of narcotic drugs is indispensable for the relief of pain and that State signatories to the treaty should take "the necessary measures to ensure the availability of narcotic drugs for such purposes."

SOMA OR CELL BODY: The area of a neuron where the cell nucleus is located and from which the dendritic projections and axon emerge.

SOMATIC-SENSORY-MOTOR CORTEX: Cortical area that includes the primary somatosensory cortex, which receives information from the skin and tongue, and the primary motor area, which sends information to the muscles.

STRIATUM OR STRIATAL SYSTEM: Set of subcortical structures involved in movement and highly related to the dopaminergic system.

SYNAPSE: An area of electrical nerve impulse transmission between two neurons, usually formed between the axon terminal of one neuron (presynaptic neuron) and the dendrite of another neuron (postsynaptic neuron).

SYNAPTIC BOUTON: Surface of the dendritic membrane that forms a protuberance where receptors for a particular synapse are localized.

SYNESTHESIA: Fusion of different senses into one.

TEMPORAL LOBE: Cerebral lobe containing the primary auditory cortex.

THALAMUS: Subcortical structure located in the centre of the brain, between the two hemispheres and just below the cerebral cortex.

TOP-DOWN INFORMATION: Information that goes from higher orders of integration to lower orders of integration. Regulates what information from lower levels reaches higher ones.

TRANSPORTERS: Proteins that allow neurotransmitters to pass through the membrane. They are located in the membranes of the axon terminal (i.e., neurotransmitter reuptake proteins) or of vesicles.

UNIÃO DO VEGETAL (UDV): Together with Santo Daime, another of the great ayahuasca churches in the world.

UNIMODAL AREA: Areas that process information from only one sense.

UNITED NATIONS COMMISSION ON NARCOTIC DRUGS (CND): Established by the Economic and Social Council (ECOSOC) of the United Nations by Resolution 9 of February 17, 1946, as the governing body of international drug control treaties. It is a functional commission of the ECOSOC. The CND meets annually in Vienna, Austria, to examine and adopt a series of decisions and resolutions related to the implementation of drug treaties and policies about narcotic drugs and psychotropic substances.

VENTRAL ATTENTIONAL NETWORK: Functional network involved in the reorientation of attention according to the personal relevance of the information in the environment. Contains the insula. Also described as the salience network.

VISUAL CORTEX: Cortical area in the occipital lobe responsible for integrating visual information.

VISUALS: Visual hallucinations induced by psychedelics that occur with the eyes closed.

VOXEL: Cubic unit that makes up a three-dimensional object. In the case of functional magnetic resonance imaging, it is the unit of measurement from which activity values are obtained over time. It usually measures three cubic millimeters.

WAR ON DRUGS: A policy promoted by the U.S. government aimed at the prosecution of the production, trade, and consumption of certain psychoactive substances. The term was popularized by the media shortly after a press conference held on June 18, 1971, by U.S. President Richard Nixon.

WORKING MEMORY: Short-term memory that allows us to maintain in our minds the informative elements needed to perform a task as we execute it.

Index